RENAL DIET PLAN & COOKBOOK

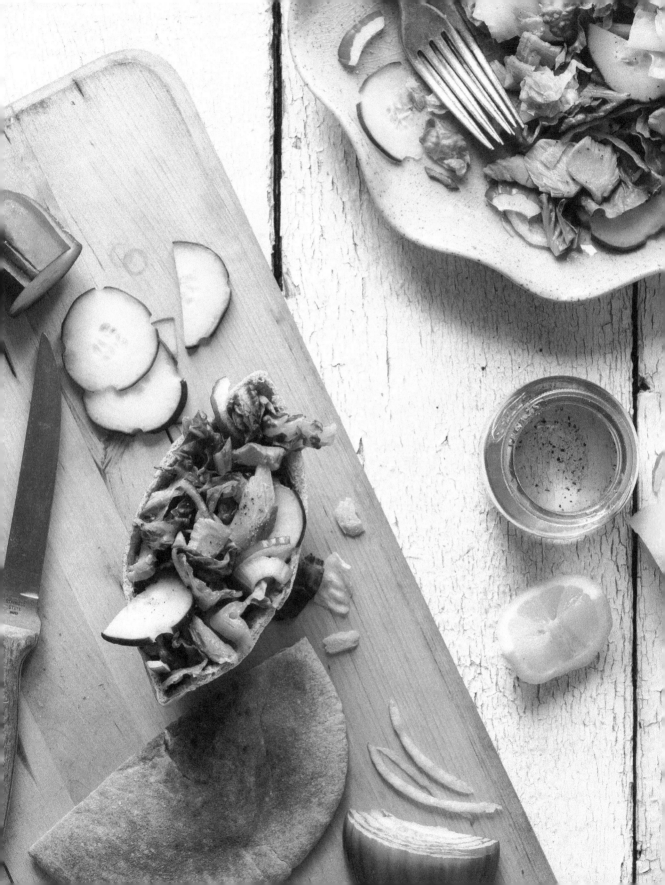

RENAL DIET PLAN & COOKBOOK

The Optimal Nutrition Guide to Manage Kidney Disease

Susan Zogheib, MHS, RD, LDN

ROCKRIDGE
PRESS

Front cover photography © 2017 Shannon Douglas

Interior photography © Stocksy/Trent Lanz, p.2; Stocksy/Trent Lanz, p.6; Stocksy/Toma Evsiukova, p.8; Stocksy/Nadine Greeff, p.14; Stockfood/Gräfe & Unzer Verlag/Anke Schütz, p.22; Stocksy/Martí Sans, p.42; Shutterstock/Evgeny Karandaev, p.46; Stockfood/Gräfe & Unzer Verlag/mona binner PHOTOGRAPHIE, p.62; Stockfood/Louise Lister, p.76; Stocksy/Harald Walker, p.88; Stockfood/Keller & Keller Photography, p.100; Stockfood/Magdalena Hendey, p.114; Stockfood/Rua Castilho, p.132; Stockfood/Great Stock!, p.148; Stocksy/Trent Lanz, p.166; Stockfood/Keller & Keller Photography, p.182; Kelly Ishikawa, p.204; Stocksy/Boris Zhuykov, p.218

Back cover photography © Stockfood/Keller & Keller Photography, Stockfood/Louise Lister, Stockfood/Magdalena Hendey

ISBN: Print 978-1-62315-869-9| eBook 978-1-62315-887-3

I dedicate this book to my beautiful nieces and nephews—Samantha, Juliana, Nicholas, Eli, Grady, and Rami. All of your dreams can come true, if you have the courage to pursue them.

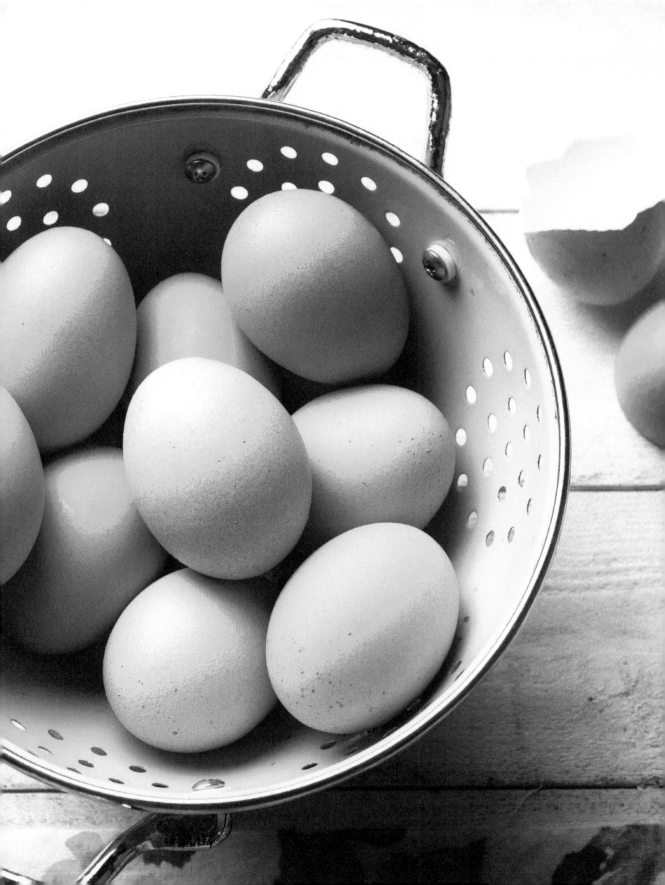

CONTENTS

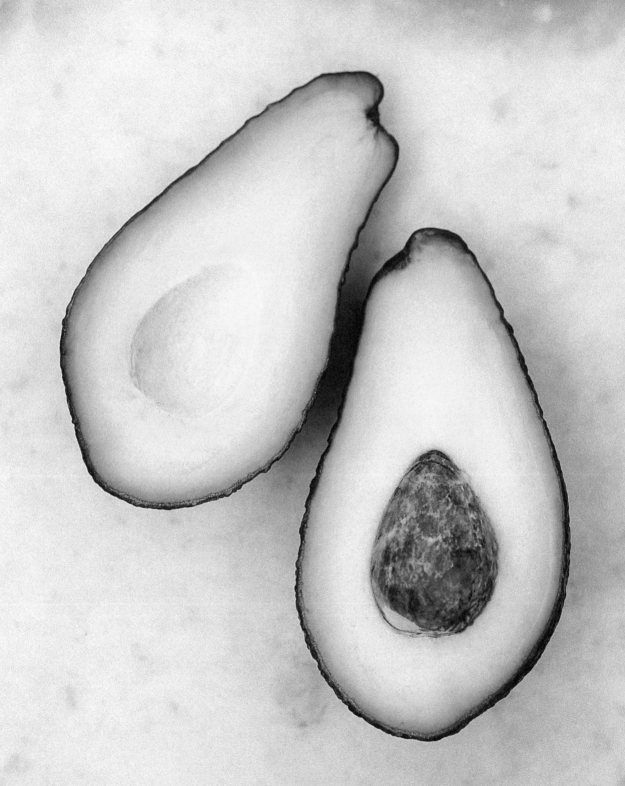

FOREWORD

The dietary and nutritional management of chronic kidney disease is one of the trickiest things we deal with as doctors. As the kidneys lose their ability to filter out waste products—along with extra fluid, sodium, potassium, and phosphorus—we tend to restrict those ingredients in our patients' diets. But at the same time, we know that too much dietary protein can make their kidney function decrease more rapidly, so we try to limit their protein, too. Also, since people with kidney disease often suffer from diabetes and heart disease, they need a diet that is lower in simple sugars, carbohydrates and fats. After we take all these things away, many patients ask, "What's left?" In the worst-case scenario, what's left is malnutrition.

The Renal Diet Plan and Cookbook, is a better answer. As an experienced dietician specializing in patients with kidney disease, Susan Zogheib explains in understandable terms how the kidneys work, how to read a nutrition label, and how to make kidney-friendly food choices. As a dietician who loves to cook, she presents easy and practical recipes that bring to life her philosophy of empowered eating and self-compassion.

My patients are tired of having doctors, nurses, and dieticians tell them what they can't do and what they can't eat. This book is a patient-centered diet plan with recipes that my patients will want to use, not just because they are kidney- and heart-healthy, but because they taste so good. Now, when my patients ask what's left, I can tell them Cobb Salad with homemade dressing, Crispy Fried Chicken, and Berry Peach Cobbler.

George R. Aronoff, MD, MS, FACP
Chief Medical Officer
Renal Ventures Management, LLC
Adjunct Professor of Medicine and Pharmacology
University of Louisville School of Medicine

INTRODUCTION

As a registered dietitian, I have worked with patients battling many health issues, including diabetes, high blood pressure, heart disease, weight management, and kidney disease. Through the years, I've noticed that patients struggling with kidney disease are often trying to manage other health conditions at the same time. If you have kidney disease, you're likely trying to also manage your blood sugar, cholesterol level, blood pressure, and weight—concurrently.

Kidney disease is a leading cause of death in the United States. But there is much we can do to treat, control, and influence the progression of kidney disease, especially in the early stages. The sooner you are diagnosed and begin responding to your special health needs, the better your kidneys can serve you. Untreated kidney disease tends to be irreversible, and puts you at a higher risk for heart disease and stroke. So it is important to identify kidney disease early. Fortunately, kidney disease can be treated effectively if it is detected in the early stages.

A key to healthier kidneys lies in your diet. I cannot overemphasize how pivotal it is to know what foods are healthier choices and which ones you should avoid—the ones that can cause more damage. A renal diet, especially in the early stages of kidney disease, focuses on limiting protein, sodium, fat, and sugar. Following a renal diet will help decrease the amount of waste made by your body, which helps your kidneys work more effectively. Even small changes in your diet can help preserve your kidney function for a long time, and may even help you avoid dialysis treatment altogether.

In my work with patients who are in the early stages of kidney disease, I've seen firsthand how they have greatly improved their kidney function simply by making the small behavioral and lifestyle changes discussed in this book, and following the renal diet provided. And by trying the delicious recipes in this book, you will discover great foods that will support your health and minimize the work your kidneys need to do to take the best care of you.

Let's get started!

PART

1

YOUR KIDNEYS, YOUR HEALTH

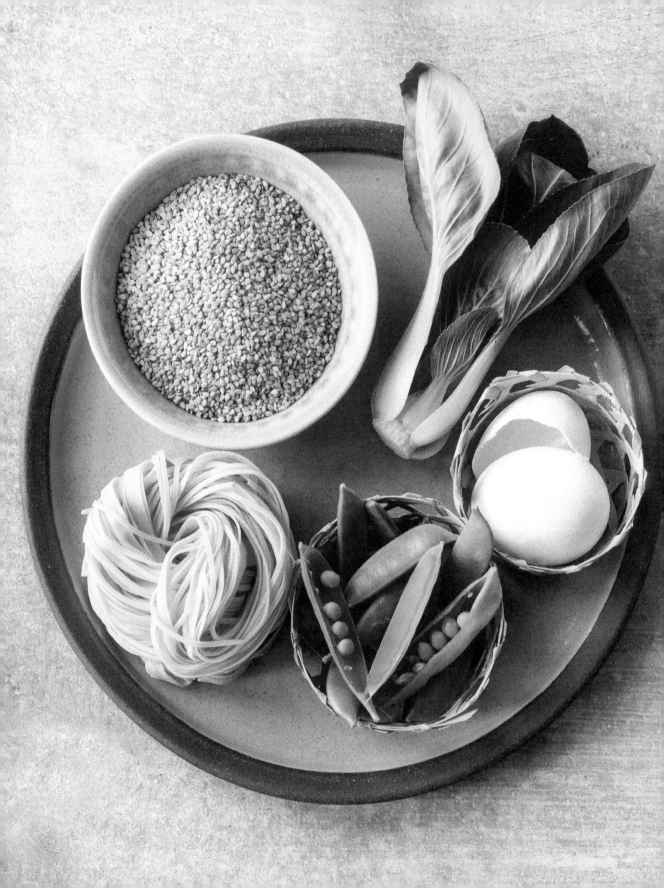

1

UNDERSTANDING KIDNEY DISEASE

Kidney disease is becoming more prevalent in the United States, and so we need to learn as much about it as we can. The more we educate ourselves, the more we can do to take care of this important bodily system. If you've been diagnosed with chronic kidney disease (CKD), education can empower you to most effectively and purposefully manage the disease. Once you have a full understanding of what chronic kidney disease is, you can begin to take charge of your evolving health needs. Making healthy changes early in the stages of kidney disease will help determine how well you will manage your kidney health. I am here to guide you, every step of the way. Like any new process, it may seem intimidating at first. But this chapter provides the foundation for learning, and will help you understand kidney disease as you begin your journey to healthier kidneys.

What Do the Kidneys Do?

Renal: *Relating to or involving the kidneys.*
—Merriam-Webster's Collegiate Dictionary

Our kidneys are small, but they do powerful things to keep our body in balance. They are bean-shaped, about the size of a fist, and are located in the middle of the back, on the left and right sides of the spine, just below the rib cage. When everything is working properly, the kidneys do many important jobs such as:

1. Filter waste materials from the blood
2. Remove extra fluid, or water, from the body
3. Release hormones that help manage blood pressure
4. Stimulate bone marrow to make red blood cells
5. Make an active form of vitamin D that promotes strong, healthy bones

Our kidneys are like a balance scale, working to keep the appropriate amounts of nutrients and minerals in the body. When the kidneys are not functioning properly, waste products and toxins will begin to accumulate in the body. Failing kidneys lose their ability to filter out waste products, resulting in kidney disease. The kidneys' inability to do their job then shifts the duty of decision to you—it becomes up to you to make changes to your diet in order to reduce the burden placed on the kidneys, especially in the early stages of kidney disease.

What Causes Kidney Disease?

There are many causes of kidney disease, including physical injury or disorders that can damage the kidneys, but the two leading causes of kidney disease are diabetes and high blood pressure. These underlying conditions also put people at risk for developing cardiovascular disease. Early treatment may not only slow down the progression of the disease, but also reduce your risk of developing heart disease or stroke.

Kidney disease can affect anyone, at any age. African Americans, Hispanics, and American Indians are at increased risk for kidney failure, because these groups have a greater prevalence of diabetes and high blood pressure.

Uncontrolled diabetes is the leading cause of kidney disease. Diabetes can damage the kidneys and cause them to fail. Diabetes is a disease in which the body does not make enough insulin or cannot use normal amounts of insulin properly, which causes blood glucose (blood sugar) levels to be high.

When we digest protein, our bodies create waste products. In the kidneys, millions of tiny blood vessels called capillaries act as filters. As blood flows through the capillaries, the waste products are filtered through the urine. Substances such as protein and red blood cells are too big to pass through the capillaries and so stay in the blood. Diabetes can damage this process, and high levels of blood sugar can make the kidneys filter too much blood. All the extra work takes a toll on the kidneys. Over time, the kidneys can start to leak, and the protein our bodies need is lost in the urine. Having small amounts of protein in your urine is called microalbuminuria. When kidney disease is detected in the early stages, several treatments may prevent the worsening of the disease. If kidney disease is detected in the later stages, high amounts of protein in your urine, called macroalbuminuria, can lead to end-stage renal disease.

The second leading cause of kidney disease is high blood pressure, also known as hypertension. One in three Americans is at risk for kidney disease because of hypertension. Although there is no cure for hypertension, certain medications, a low-sodium diet, and physical activity can lower blood pressure.

The kidneys help manage blood pressure, but when blood pressure is high, the heart has to work overtime at pumping blood. High blood pressure can damage the blood vessels in the kidneys, reducing their ability to work efficiently. When the force of blood flow is high, blood vessels start to stretch so the blood can flow more easily. The stretching and scarring weakens the blood vessels throughout the entire body, including the kidneys. And when the kidneys' blood vessels are injured, they may not remove the waste and extra fluid from the body, creating a dangerous cycle, because the extra fluid in the blood vessels can increase blood pressure even more.

Cardiovascular disease is the leading cause of death in the United States. The heart does an extraordinary job at pumping oxygen and nutrient-rich blood through our arteries to vital organs—including the brain—and tissues. When kidney disease occurs, that process can be affected, and the risk of developing heart disease becomes greater. Cardiovascular disease is an umbrella term used to describe conditions that may damage the heart and blood vessels, including coronary artery disease, heart attack, heart failure, atherosclerosis, and high blood pressure. Complications from renal disease may develop, and can lead to heart disease.

With diabetes, excess blood sugar remains in the bloodstream. The high blood sugar levels can damage the blood vessels in the kidneys and elsewhere in the body. And since high blood pressure is a complication from diabetes, the extra pressure can weaken the walls of the blood vessels, which can lead to a heart attack or stroke.

Other conditions, such as drug abuse and certain autoimmune diseases, can also cause injury to the kidneys. In fact, every drug we put into our body has to pass through the kidneys for filtration. If the drug is not taken following a healthcare provider's instructions, or if it is an illegal substance such as heroin, cocaine, or ecstasy, it can cause injury to the kidneys by raising the blood pressure, also increasing the risk of a stroke, heart failure, and even death.

An autoimmune disease is one in which the immune system, designed to protect the body from illness, sees the body as an invader and attacks its own systems, including the kidneys. Some forms of lupus, for example, attack the kidneys. Another autoimmune disease that can lead to kidney failure is Goodpasture syndrome, a group of conditions that affect the kidneys and the lungs. The damage to the kidneys from autoimmune diseases can lead to chronic kidney disease and kidney failure.

TREATMENT PLANS FOR CHRONIC KIDNEY DISEASE (CKD)

The best way to manage CKD is to be an active participant in your treatment program, regardless of your stage of renal disease. Proper treatment involves a combination of working with a healthcare team, adhering to a renal diet, and making healthy lifestyle decisions. These can all have a profoundly positive effect on your kidney disease—especially watching how you eat.

Working with your healthcare team. When you have kidney disease, working in partnership with your healthcare team can be extremely important in your treatment program as well as being personally empowering. Regularly meeting with your physician or healthcare team can arm you with resources and information that help you make informed decisions regarding your treatment needs, and provide you with a much needed opportunity to vent, share information, get advice, and receive support in effectively managing this illness.

Adhering to a renal diet. The heart of this book is the renal diet. Sticking to this diet can make a huge difference in your health and vitality. Like any change, following the diet may not be easy at first. Important changes to your diet, particularly early on, can possibly prevent the need for dialysis. These changes include limiting salt, eating a low-protein diet, reducing fat intake, and getting enough calories if you need to lose weight. Be honest with yourself first and foremost—learn what you need, and consider your personal goals and obstacles. Start by making small changes. It is okay to have some slip-ups—we all do. With guidance and support, these small changes will become habits of your promising new lifestyle. In no time, you will begin taking control of your diet and health.

Making healthy lifestyle decisions. Lifestyle choices play a crucial part in our health, especially when it comes to helping regulate kidney disease. Lifestyle choices such as allotting time for physical activity, getting enough sleep, managing weight, reducing stress, and limiting smoking and alcohol will help you take control of your overall health, making it easier to manage your kidney disease. Follow this simple formula: Keep toxins out of your body as much as you can, and build up your immune system with a good balance of exercise, relaxation, and sleep.

What are the Symptoms of Kidney Disease?

Some people in the early stages of kidney disease may not even show any symptoms. If you suffer from diabetes or high blood pressure, it is important to manage it early on in order to protect your kidneys. Although kidney failure occurs over the course of many years, you may not show any signs until kidney disease or failure has occurred.

When the kidneys are damaged, wastes and toxins can build up in the body, because the kidneys are not able to filter them as effectively. Once this buildup begins, you may start to feel sick and experience some of the following symptoms:

- Anemia (low red blood cell count)
- Blood in urine
- Bone pain
- Difficulty concentrating
- Difficulty sleeping
- Dry and itchy skin
- Muscle cramps (especially in the legs)
- Nausea
- Poor appetite
- Swelling in feet and ankles
- Tiredness
- Weakness
- Weight loss

Fortunately, once treatment for kidney disease begins, especially if caught in the early stages, symptoms tend to lessen and general health will begin to improve.

The Five Stages of Chronic Kidney Disease

Chronic kidney disease is categorized by five stages, as shown in the following table. Each stage of kidney disease is identified by the presence of kidney damage and the decrease of glomerular filtration rate (GFR), which measure the effectiveness of kidney function. Treatment varies depending on the stage of kidney disease. Stage 1 is the earliest stage; it is reflective of generally good kidney function but perhaps some visible inflammation or anomaly of the kidney, and/or protein or blood in the urine. Stage 5 is considered kidney failure, usually signifying the need for dialysis or a kidney transplant. Signs and symptoms develop more rapidly with the disease's progression through the different stages. Consult your doctor if you have any questions about your stage of kidney disease or treatment.

Five Stages of Chronic Kidney Disease

STAGE	DESCRIPTION	GLOMERULAR FILTRATION RATE (GFR)
Normal kidney function	Healthy kidneys	90 mL/min or more
Stage 1	Kidney damage with normal or high GFR	90 mL/min or more
Stage 2	Kidney damage with mild decrease in GFR	60–89 mL/min
Stage 3	Moderate decrease in GFR	30–59 mL/min
Stage 4	Severe decrease in GFR	15–29 mL/min
Stage 5	Kidney failure	Less than 15 mL/min or receiving dialysis

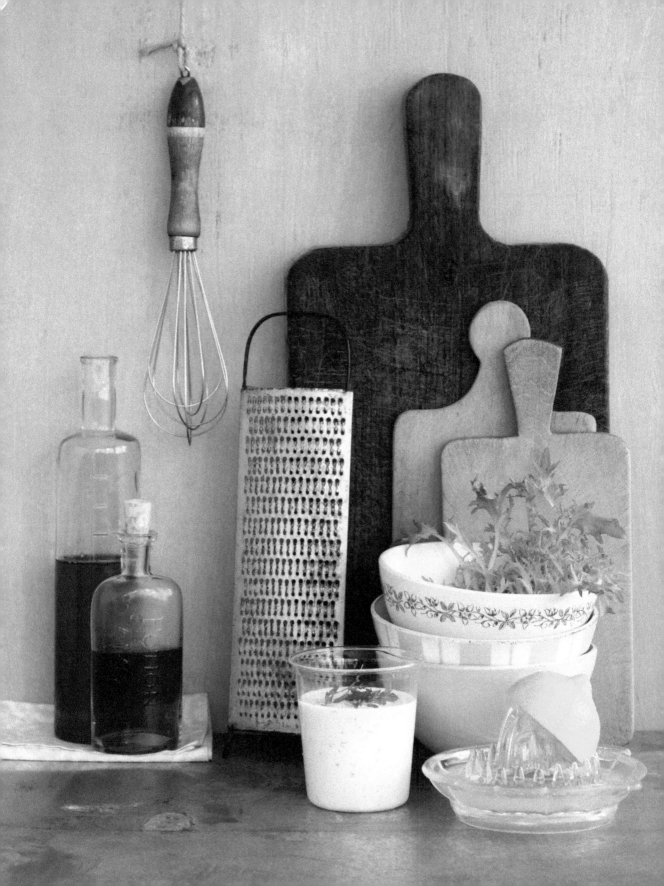

2

EMPOWERED EATING
FOR HEALTHIER LIVING

In this chapter, we'll explore what healthy eating really means. At first it may seem overwhelming, but stick with me—you'll see it's pretty simple and can even be fun. And as you build your awareness of what you're putting into your body, you may find yourself increasingly passionate about nutrition, and eager to try all the foods that are delicious *and* good for you. By the end of this chapter, you will have all the tools to get you started. Just be open-minded, and try not to be too hard on yourself. You may have some days when you are not up for eating healthy, and it's okay. We all have a bad day here and there. But your new knowledge will help direct you. I will show you how to read nutrition labels with a critical eye, and empower you to make healthier choices that will help your kidneys thrive, without leaving you feeling deprived.

A Commitment to Healthy Eating

There's no place like home. Cooking healthy homemade meals from simple, easily identifiable ingredients will help you manage the condition of your kidneys and slow the progression of the disease. Our modern age has affected our diets, and not in a good way. Fewer people are cooking, and more are turning to fast food. For many, sitting down to a nutritious meal together is a thing of the past. We're constantly on the go, and seek easy and quick fixes to get us through the day. The more processed foods we consume, the less we are aware of what is in the food itself. Last-minute take-out or packaged dinners are often loaded with calories, fats, sodium, preservatives, and added sweeteners—none of which are beneficial for the body, and all of which can harm your kidneys or hasten the progression of CKD. The single greatest change you can make for your health is in your diet: healthy eating truly matters. It is never too late to start making a positive effect on your health.

Key Nutritional Concerns

When you have kidney disease, you may also be trying to manage your high blood pressure, heart disease, and/or diabetes. While there is no one eating plan that is perfect for everyone with kidney disease, following this renal diet with any necessary modifications based on your individual restrictions will help keep your kidneys as healthy as possible. Your particular eating plan will also depend on your stage of kidney disease, since what you can or cannot eat may change over time. Generally, however, the renal diet presented in this book will lay the foundation by providing you with delicious, kidney-friendly recipes. Here are some key nutrients I would like you to focus on—some you need more of, and others less. Knowing more about them is important to kidney health.

Phosphorus

This mineral can be found in every cell of our bodies, but mostly in the teeth and bones—it provides structural support to DNA and RNA. Phosphorus also helps us filter waste from the kidneys, but interestingly, too much phosphorus can be detrimental in CKD. Healthy kidneys can filter excess phosphorus and other waste from the body, but during early stage kidney disease, the kidneys must work harder to remove it. In fact, studies reveal that reducing phosphorus intake in earlier stages of CKD may help maintain kidney function as well as healthy bones and a healthy heart.

For people with CKD and those receiving dialysis, phosphorus in the diet should be restricted to between 800 and 1,000 milligrams per day. As kidney function diminishes, extra phosphorus can start building up in the blood, causing the bones to get weaker. Talk with your dietitian or healthcare provider, who can tell you if you need to limit foods that are high in phosphorus, and/or prescribe a phosphate binder to help control your phosphorus levels.

Phosphorus in Common Foods*

LOW PHOSPHORUS (Less than 150 mg/serving)	MEDIUM PHOSPHORUS (151–250 mg/serving)	HIGH PHOSPHORUS (More than 251 mg/serving)
Apple	Beans, black, 1 cup	Peanuts, oil roasted, 2 ounces
Bagel, 1 plain (4-inch diameter)	Beans, fava, 1 cup	Almonds, oil/dry roasted, 2 ounces
Barley, pearled, cooked	Beans, kidney, 1 cup	Baked beans, 1 cup
Beans, green	Beans, pinto, 1 cup	Beans, small white, mature, boiled, 1 cup
Bread, pita, 1 (6.5-inch diameter)	Beef, bottom round, 3 ounces	Beef, liver, cooked, 3 ounces
Bread, pumpernickel, 2 slices	Beef, chuck roast, 3 ounces	Beefalo, 3 ounces
Bread, white, 2 slices	Beef, eye round, 3 ounces	Buttermilk, 1 cup
Butter, 1 tablespoon	Beef, ground, 70% lean, 3 ounces	Calamari, fried, 3 ounces
	Beef, ground, 95% lean, 3 ounces	

*One serving = ½ cup unless otherwise noted. ▶

Phosphorus in Common Foods*

LOW PHOSPHORUS (Less than 150 mg/serving)	MEDIUM PHOSPHORUS (151–250 mg/serving)	HIGH PHOSPHORUS (More than 251 mg/serving)
Cabbage	Beef, sirloin steak, 3 ounces	Cashews, dry roasted, 2 ounces
Cauliflower	Black-eyed peas, 1 cup	Cereal, bran, 100%
Cereal, crispy rice, 1 cup	Bread, whole wheat, 2 slices	Cereal, wheat germ, ¼ cup
Cheese, Brie, 1 ounce	Catfish, breaded/fried, 3 ounces	Cheese, goat, 2 ounces
Cheese, feta, 1 ounce	Cheese, blue, 2 ounces	Cheese, Parmesan, 2 ounces
Cocoa, unsweetened, 2 tablespoons	Cheese, Cheddar, 1 ounce	Cheese, ricotta, part skim
Cookies, shortbread, 4	Cheese, mozzarella, 1 ounce	Cheese, Romano, 2 ounces
Cornflakes, 1 cup	Cheese, provolone, 2 ounces	Chia seeds, 1 ounce
Cottage cheese, nonfat	Cheese, Swiss, 1 ounce	Chicken, liver, cooked, 3 ounces
Couscous, cooked	Chicken, breast, 3 ounces	Clam chowder, New England
Cream cheese, 1 ounce	Chicken, dark meat, 3 ounces	Clams, cooked with moist heat, 3 ounces
Cucumber	Chickpeas, 1 cup	Corn bread, 1 piece
Duck, with skin, 3 ounces	Chocolate, plain, 2 ounces	Crab, Alaska king, cooked with moist heat, 3 ounces
Egg white, 1 large	Cod, Pacific, 3 ounces	Custard, flan, 1 cup
Egg yolk, 1 large	Cottage cheese, 1% fat	Flounder, 3 ounces
Eggplant	Cottage cheese, 2% fat	Halibut, Atlantic/Pacific, 3 ounces
English muffin, 1 plain	Crab, blue, cooked with moist heat, 3 ounces	Lentils, mature, boiled, 1 cup
Figs	Crab, Dungeness, cooked with moist heat, 3 ounces	Milk, 1%, 1 cup
Gelatin, water base	Lamb, kabobs, domestic, 3 ounces	Milk, chocolate, 1 cup
Ginger ale, 1 can	Lamb, leg roast, domestic, 3 ounces	Milk, evaporated, nonfat
Grapefruit	Lamb, New Zealand, 3 ounces	Milk, nonfat, 1 cup
Grapes	Lobster, cooked with moist heat, 3 ounces	Milk, whole, 1 cup
Grouper		Mussels, blue, cooked with moist heat, 3 ounces
Hominy grits		Nuts, Brazil, 2 ounces
Ice cream, 10% fat, vanilla		Nuts, pine, 2 ounces
Lettuce		
Milk, soy, 1 cup		
Oatmeal, cooked, 1 packet		

*One serving = ½ cup unless otherwise noted.

Phosphorus in Common Foods*

LOW PHOSPHORUS (Less than 150 mg/serving)	MEDIUM PHOSPHORUS (151–250 mg/serving)	HIGH PHOSPHORUS (More than 251 mg/serving)
Onions	Macadamia nuts, 3 ounces	Oysters, Eastern, cooked with moist heat, 3 ounces
Oysters, canned, 3 ounces	Milk, canned, sweetened, condensed, ¼ cup	Peanuts, boiled, 1 cup
Oysters, raw, Pacific, 3 ounces	Mushrooms, cooked, 1 cup	Peanuts, dry roasted, 3 ounces
Pasta, 1 cup	Mussels, raw, blue, 3 ounces	Peanuts, oil roasted, 2 ounces
Peas, split, mature, boiled	Peanut butter, 2 tablespoons	Pecans, oil/dry roasted, 3 ounces
Plums	Pork, boneless loin chop, 3 ounces	Salmon, canned, pink/red, 3 ounces
Popcorn, air-popped, 1 cup	Pork, leg roast, 3 ounces	Sardines, canned in oil, 3 ounces
Pork, spare ribs, 3 ounces	Raisin Bran, 1 cup	Scallops, breaded/fried, 3 ounces
Radishes	Raisins, seedless, 1 cup	Sole, 3 ounces
Rice cakes, 1 cake	Rice, brown, cooked, 1 cup	Soybeans, mature, boiled
Rice, white, enriched, cooked	Shredded Wheat, 1 cup	Sunflower seeds, 1 ounce
Sherbet	Shrimp, breaded/fried, 3 ounces	Swordfish, 3 ounces
Shrimp, cooked with moist heat, 3 ounces	Snapper, 3 ounces	Tofu, raw, firm
Sour cream	Spinach, raw	Tuna, light, canned in oil, 3 ounces
Tofu, soft	Tortilla, 2 corn or flour (6-inch diameter)	Tuna, white, canned in oil, 3 ounces
Wheat flour, white, 1 cup	Turkey, breast, 3 ounces	Veal, cubed, stewed, 3 ounces
	Turkey, dark meat, 3 ounces	Walnuts, English, 2 ounces
	Veal, rib roast, 3 ounces	Wheat flour, whole grain, 1 cup
	Wheat flakes, 1 cup	Yogurt, low-fat
		Yogurt, skim

*One serving = ½ cup unless otherwise noted.

Protein

Protein plays an important role in the body, and is crucial to staying healthy. It allows your body to counteract everyday wear and tear, heal from injury, stop bleeding, and fight infections. However, too much protein can put a strain on your kidneys, and even cause additional damage. You can talk with your healthcare provider about how a reduced protein diet may help slow the progression of CKD. If you're in the early stages of chronic kidney disease, such as stages 1 and 2, your protein intake will be limited to 12 to 15 percent of your calorie intake each day, which is the same level recommended by the Dietary Reference Intakes (DRIs) for a healthy diet for normal adults. For example, if you are following a 2,000-calorie diet, your protein intake should be limited to 60 to 75 grams of protein (see Calculate Your Intake, page 30). People receiving dialysis should take in about 1.2 grams of protein per kilogram of body weight each day (1 kilogram is about 2.2 pounds). For those in stages 3 and 4, recommended protein intake is between 0.6 and 0.75 g/kg, according to the Kidney Disease Outcomes Quality Initiative (KDOQI) of The National Kidney Foundation.

As you choose your protein sources, it's important to know that some foods contain more useful and healthy proteins than others. See Low-Protein Foods (page 29) for a detailed list.

Fats

People with kidney disease are at an increased risk for developing heart disease. If your blood lipid (fat) levels are high, you may need to cut down on the amount of fat you eat. When your risk increases for heart disease, you can develop other problems such as diabetes and high blood pressure. But today we know more than ever before about health-supportive options. Vegetable fats like olive oil or canola oil are the healthiest to use in cooking. In the early stages of CKD, your blood potassium and blood phosphorus levels may also be low enough so you can enjoy avocados, nuts, and seeds in your diet, as sources for healthy fats. Tuna and salmon also contain heart-healthy fats that make a good addition to your diet. The key is to keep your fat intake to less than 30 percent of your daily calories. For example, if your caloric allowance is 2,000 calories, your calories from fat should be limited to 600 calories, or about 70 grams of fat (see Calculate Your Intake, page 30).

Low-Protein Foods

SEAFOOD, MEAT, AND POULTRY*	VEGETABLES, LEGUMES, AND NUTS**	BREADS, CEREALS, AND GRAINS***	DAIRY, EGGS, AND TOFU****
Beef	Beans, canned	Bagel, ½	Cheese (hard cheeses such as Cheddar, mozzarella, Swiss, Gouda, Colby), 1 ounce
Chicken	Beans, green and wax	Bread, 1 slice	
Clams, 5 small or 2 large	Broccoli	Biscuit or roll, 1	Cream (coffee cream, half-and-half)
Fish	Cabbage, green and red	Bun (hamburger or roll), ½	Cream soups
Lamb	Carrots	Cereals, cold (Cheerios, corn flakes, puffed rice), 1 cup	Cottage cheese, ¼ cup
Shrimp or scallops, 4	Cauliflower		
Pork	Celery	Cereals, hot (oatmeal, grits, rice, Cream of Wheat/ farina), ½ cup	Eggs or egg substitute, 1 medium or ¼ cup
Tuna or salmon, ⅛ cup or 1 ounce	Coleslaw		
Turkey	Cucumbers	Cornbread, homemade, one 2-inch cube	Ice cream
	Eggplant		Milk, whole, 2%, 1%, fat-free (skim), soy milk
	Escarole	Crackers (unsalted or graham crackers), 10	
	Greens, mustard, turnip	Muffin, homemade, 1	Pudding and custard
	Lettuce	Pancakes or waffles, homemade, 1 (4-inch diameter)	Tofu, ¼ cup
	Peanut butter or nut butters, 2 tablespoons		Yogurt, plain
	Peas, green, canned	Pasta or rice, cooked ½ cup	
		Pita bread pocket, ½	
		Popcorn (unsalted), 2 cups	
		Tortilla, 1	

* One serving = 1 ounce, providing about 7 grams of protein unless otherwise noted.

** One serving = ½ cup, providing about 2 grams of protein unless otherwise noted.

*** One serving = varies by food, providing about 2 to 3 grams of protein.

**** One serving = ½ cup, providing about 4 to 6 grams of protein unless otherwise noted.

CALCULATE YOUR INTAKE!

Do you want to learn more about the foods you are putting in your body? Visit webmd.com/diet/food-calculator. This valuable tool can help you determine calories, calories from fat, and nutritional content. Over time, you'll know where your new favorite foods stand without even checking!

Sodium

Sodium is an important mineral that helps regulate your body's water content and blood pressure. Sodium is also a major electrolyte, which helps control the fluid in the body's tissues and cells. When your kidneys are working the way they are supposed to, they can remove sodium from the body as needed. However, much like phosphorus, when your kidneys are not working properly the sodium build up in your body and make your blood pressure rise, make you thirsty, and result in water retention, causing you to gain weight.

For people in the early stages of chronic kidney disease—stages 1, 2, or 3— it is suggested that you restrict your sodium intake to between 2,000 mg and 3,000 mg per day (See Calculate Your Intake, above). If you have stage 4 or 5 chronic kidney disease and require dialysis, even lower amounts may be prescribed. It is recommended that you consume no more than 1,500 mg of sodium each day.

Carbohydrates and Fiber

We hear a lot about "carbs"—some good, some bad. Carbohydrates are necessary for fueling our body. Besides providing energy, foods rich in carbohydrates often contain vitamins, minerals, fiber, and other compounds that help protect the body. But not just any carb will do. In your journey to good health, look for carbohydrates that contain fiber (see High-Fiber Foods, below). Fiber is a nondigestible material, helping move other foods through your digestive system. It also protects your heart, blood vessels, and colon. Since people with CKD are more susceptible to heart disease, high-fiber diets are especially valuable in helping lower cholesterol levels, which reduces the risk for heart attack or other cardiovascular conditions. Fiber can help control your weight and blood sugar levels. The recommended amount of fiber for people with chronic kidney disease and on dialysis is at least 25 grams per day. So get friendly with your fiber!

High-Fiber Foods*

FRUITS (1–4g fiber)	VEGETABLES (1–4g fiber)	BREADS AND GRAINS (1–6g fiber)
Apple, raw with skin, 2.5 grams	Asparagus, 1.4 grams	Air-popped popcorn, 1 cup, 1.2 grams
Applesauce, 3 grams	Beans, green/yellow, 3.4 grams	Barley, pearled, cooked, 6 grams
Apricot, halves, 1.5 grams	Broccoli, 1.1 grams	Bread, white, 2 slices, 1.6 grams
Blackberries, 4 grams	Cabbage, raw, 1.1 grams	Corn grits, yellow, cooked, 1 cup, 1 gram
Blueberries, 1.8 grams	Carrots, 1.8 grams	
Pear, raw with skin, 3 grams	Cauliflower, cooked, 1 gram	Cornflakes, 1 cup, 1 gram
Raspberries, 4 grams	Corn, cooked, 1.8 grams	Flaxseed, whole, 1 tablespoon, 2.8 grams
Strawberries, sliced, 1.7 grams	Peas, frozen, cooked, 4 grams	Grape-Nuts Flakes, ¾ cup, 3 grams
Tangerine, 1.8 grams	Zucchini, cooked, 1 cup, 1.8 grams	Rice, brown, cooked, 1.7 grams

*One serving = ½ cup unless otherwise noted.

Potassium

Potassium is a mineral and electrolyte that regulates metabolism and fluid levels and helps your muscles, kidneys, and heart function properly, but only in the right doses—it depends on how well your kidneys are working and whether you are taking medications that affect potassium levels. In the early stages of kidney disease, potassium levels are usually normal. If your potassium level is above normal during stages 1, 2, or 3 of CKD, your physician will probably conduct a blood test to help determine the cause and whether you need to make any dietary changes. If you are receiving dialysis, your potassium intake should be limited to 2,000 to 3,000 milligrams per day (see Calculate Your Intake, page 30). Excess potassium can harm the heart muscle and cause an irregular heartbeat or difficulty breathing, so maintaining the right balance is essential.

Potassium in Common Foods*

LOW POTASSIUM (Less than 150 mg/serving)	MEDIUM POTASSIUM (151–250 mg/serving)	HIGH POTASSIUM (More than 251 mg/serving)
Alfalfa seeds, sprouted, raw	Apple, without skin, 1 large	Apricot, 1 cup
Apple juice	Apricot, halves, 1 medium	Artichoke, 1 medium
Applesauce, sweetened	Apricots, in heavy syrup, drained	Avocado
Bagel, 1 plain (4-inch diameter)	Asparagus, boiled, 5 spears	Bamboo shoots, cooked
Beans, green, frozen	Beans, green, boiled, 1 cup	Banana, 1 small
Blueberries	Blackberries, 1 cup	Beans, black, mature, boiled
Cabbage, shredded, boiled	Broccoli, frozen, 1 cup	Beans, dried
Carrot, baby raw, 1 medium	Brussels sprouts, boiled	Beans, Lima, large, mature, boiled, ⅓ cup
Cherries, sour canned, in syrup	Carrots, sliced, 1 cup	Beans, pinto, mature, boiled
Coffee, 1 cup	Cereal, All-Bran	Beans, refried, canned
Cranberries, dried	Cherries, 10 sweet	Beets, cooked
Cranberry juice	Chickpeas, dried, boiled	Cabbage, Chinese, cooked
Cranberry sauce, canned	Collards, chopped, frozen	Cantaloupe, cubed, 1 cup
	Corn, yellow, boiled, 1 ear	Chard, Swiss, boiled, ⅓ cup

*One serving = ½ cup unless otherwise noted.

LOW POTASSIUM (Less than 150 mg/serving)	MEDIUM POTASSIUM (151–250 mg/serving)	HIGH POTASSIUM (More than 251 mg/serving)
Eggplant, boiled	Date, dried, 1 date	Chocolate
Fig, raw, 1 medium	Elderberries	Dates, Medjool
Ginger ale, 12 ounces	Grapefruit, ½ medium	Fruits, dried
Grapes	Grapefruit juice	Mango, pieces, 1 cup
Lemon, 1 medium	Grape juice, 1 cup	Milk, 1%, 1 cup
Lime, 1 medium	Honeydew melon, pieces	Milk, soy, 1 cup
Mustard greens, frozen	Kiwifruit, 1 medium	Milk, whole, 1 cup
Oatmeal, regular	Leeks, 1 raw	Molasses, 1 tablespoon
Okra, cooked	Mustard greens, cooked, ¾ cup	Mushrooms, cooked, 1 cup
Onions, raw, diced		Nectarine, 1 medium
Parsley, raw, 10 sprigs	Onion, chopped, boiled	Nuts, mixed, 2 ounces
Peaches, canned, in syrup, drained	Orange, 1 medium	Orange juice, fresh
	Peach, 1 small	Papaya, 1 small
Pears, canned, in syrup, drained	Pear, 1 medium	Plantain, sliced, cooked
	Peppers, hot chile	Pomegranate, 1 small
Peppers, sweet, cooked	Peppers, sweet, raw	Pomegranate juice
Pineapple, pieces	Pineapple, canned	Potatoes, white, baked, 1 medium
Plum, 1 medium	Pineapple juice	
Popcorn, buttered	Prickly pear, 1 medium	Raisins, seedless, 1.5-ounce box
Prunes, dried, 1 prune	Prunes, canned, 5 prunes	
Radicchio, raw, shredded	Radishes, raw, sliced, 1 cup	Sapodilla, 1 medium
Raspberries	Raspberries, frozen, sweetened, 1 cup	Sauerkraut, undrained, 1 cup
Rhubarb, cooked with sugar		Spinach, cooked
Rice, white, enriched, 1 cup cooked	Scallions, chopped, raw, 1 cup	Succotash, boiled
	Squash, summer	Sweet potatoes, boiled
Spaghetti, enriched, cooked	Strawberries, whole, 1 cup	Tomato, 1 medium
Spinach, raw, chopped	Tangerine, 1 large	Tomato paste, canned, ¼ cup
Tea, black, 8 ounces	Tortillas, corn, 4 (6-inch diameter)	Tomato sauce, canned, ¼ cup
Turnips, white, cubed		
Water chestnuts, canned	Turnip greens, chopped	Water chestnuts, raw
Watermelon, pieces		

*One serving = ½ cup unless otherwise noted.

HOW TO READ A FOOD NUTRITION FACTS LABEL

Most packaged food products have a food nutrition facts label. To make healthier choices, it is helpful, even eye-opening, to understand how to read a food label. Follow the tips below for making the most of the information on the label:

1.

2.

3.

4.

5.

Nutrition Facts

Serving Size 1 cup (110g)
Servings Per Container About 6

Amount Per Serving

Calories 250   Calories from Fat 30

	% Daily Value*
Total Fat 7g	**11%**
Saturated Fat 3g	**16%**
Trans Fat 0g	
Cholesterol 4mg	**2%**
Sodium 300mg	**13%**
Total Carbohydrate 30g	**10%**
Dietary Fiber 3g	**14%**
Sugars 2g	
Protein 5g	
Vitamin A	7%
Vitamin C	15%
Calcium	20%
Iron	32%

* Percent Daily Values are based on a 2,000 calorie diet. Your daily value may be higher or lower depending on your calorie needs.

	Calories:	2,000	2,500
Total Fat	Less than	55g	75g
Saturated Fat	Less than	10g	12g
Cholesterol	Less than	1,500mg	1,700mg
Total Carbohydrate		250mg	300mg
Dietary Fiber		22mg	31mg

1. **Start at the top of the label with the serving information.**

This will tell you the size of a single serving and the total number of servings per container (package). For example, one serving for this product is 1 cup. You may be surprised by looking at the label to see that your favorite processed food snack is not really one serving, but perhaps two or three!

2. **Next, let's check the total calories per serving.**

A 1-cup serving of this food product has 250 calories. Be careful to pay attention to the calories per serving so you do not eat too much of a product. If you double the servings you eat, you double the calories and nutrients—in this case, you would have consumed 500 calories.

3. **Limit some nutrients.**

Based on a 2,000-calorie diet per day, the American Heart Association (AHA) recommends the average person consume no more than 11 to 13 grams of saturated fat, as little trans fat as possible, and no more than 1,500 mg of sodium. These guidelines may vary if you are on a renal diet; your healthcare provider can guide you.

4. **Get plenty of these nutrients.**

These nutrients listed on the label will benefit your body on a daily basis: dietary fiber, protein, calcium, iron, and vitamins and minerals. We'll go more into depth on which ones you may need to watch, and your healthcare provider can also help provide healthy guidelines.

5. **Make the most of % Daily Value.**

The % Daily Value (DV) shows the percentage of a nutrient in a serving as it pertains to the daily recommended amount. According to the American Heart Association, to consume less of a nutrient (such as sodium), look for foods with a lower % DV (the AHA recommends 5 percent or less). If you want to consume more of a nutrient, look for foods with a higher % DV (the AHA recommends 20 percent or more).

Vitamin and Mineral Supplements

Vitamins and minerals are substances your body needs to help carry out specialized functions. They help your body use the foods you eat. Vitamins and minerals provide you with energy, help your body grow and repair tissue, and maintain life. Everyone needs them. But if you have kidney disease and/or are on dialysis, you may need to supplement some of them.

If you have kidney disease or are receiving dialysis, avoid over-the-counter multivitamins. Vitamins A, E, and K should be limited or avoided, because levels of these vitamins build up in the body as kidney function decreases. Focus on B complex vitamins and folic acid—these do not accumulate in the body and must be replaced daily, so you need more of them. If you have anemia, you may need to take an iron supplement to boost red blood cell production. Talk with your physician about the best supplemental options for you, such as getting a prescription for a renal multivitamin.

Fluids

Most people in the early stages of kidney disease do not need to limit the amount of fluids they drink. When kidney function slows down, the kidneys will produce less urine. The less urine your kidneys make, the less fluid you should drink. The daily amount of fluid you are allowed to drink depends on the amount of urine you produce.

A fluid is any food or beverage that turns to liquid at room temperature. It includes water and ice cubes, tea, coffee, soft drinks, juice, milk and milk products, gravy, sauces, soups, ice cream, jelly and gelatin, custard, and yogurt.

Drinking too much fluid can result in fluid retention, which can lead to high blood pressure and edema (swelling), and it may cause congestive heart failure. In early stages of CKD (stages 1 through 4), you do not need to limit your fluid intake as long as your urine output is normal. In stage 5, you may have to restrict your fluid intake. For people receiving dialysis, liquids are usually limited to 32 to 48 ounces (1,000 to 1,500 milliliters) per day.

Calories

Caloric requirements vary from person to person. Everyone needs calories; they give us energy for everyday life. If you don't get enough calories, your body will use protein from your muscles for energy, making you weak and potentially damaging your kidneys. Getting the right number of calories is also important for maintaining a healthy weight. If your caloric intake is too high, you will likely gain weight, which can also burden the kidneys.

Whether you are on dialysis or not, caloric requirements for anyone with CKD are 30 to 35 calories per kilogram of body weight. If you weigh 150 pounds, this equates to about 2,000 calories per day.

Healthy Cooking Techniques

Following a renal diet does not mean you have to sacrifice all the good stuff. With a little inspiration and maybe a little tweak to your cooking style, you can still enjoy your favorite foods that are packed with plenty of flavor. You'll learn about healthy cooking methods that will help you cut down on added salt and fat. Here are some healthier cooking techniques to make your time in the kitchen rewarding to both your palate and your body:

Baking Baking or roasting food uses prolonged dry heat, normally in an oven. It cooks from all sides at once. This smart cooking option for meats and vegetables results in crispy outsides and tender insides.

Broiling Broiling entails cooking food under high, direct heat for a short period of time, which is especially useful for cooking tender cuts of meat. For a healthy option, trim the excess fat around the meat before cooking.

Grilling Grilling is a great cooking method to maximize nutrition without sacrificing flavor. It uses minimal added fats and provides a smoky flavor while keeping meats and vegetables juicy and tender.

Poaching Poaching means cooking a food in a small amount of hot liquid such as water, milk, or wine (just below boiling point). This technique gently cooks delicate foods like fish, eggs, or fruit.

Steaming Steaming allows a food to cook above liquid so it cooks in its own juices and retains all its nutrients. You can steam anything from fresh vegetables to fish fillets. To enhance flavor, you may want to add a little seasoning to the food item first, such as a mixture of spices or a squeeze of lemon juice.

Stir-frying Stir-frying is creative, versatile, and fun. This method requires some oil in the pan, but only a small amount—just enough to get a nice sear on your meat and veggies. Stir-frying is very effective for bite-size pieces of meat, grains like rice and quinoa, and thinly cut veggies such as sliced bell peppers, julienned carrots, and sliced snow peas.

Practicing Self-Compassion

During another long day at work, you realize you forgot to eat lunch. You're starving. You can hear your stomach growling, "Feed me." The salad you brought that day doesn't look so good anymore. Your coworker offers to share the pizza she ordered. Who doesn't love pizza? So you take a slice, eating it quickly because you're so hungry. Minutes pass and you're feeling guilty about your choice, so you take another slice thinking to yourself at that point you really messed up your diet—but it was soooo good. So you take another slice. You're left feeling full to the point of busting and you start criticizing yourself for your lack of willpower. "I shouldn't have eaten that. What's wrong with me? Why can't I control my actions?" It happens to all of us. It's especially common for those who try without success to eat more healthily by depriving themselves of foods they enjoy, only to overindulge later.

Instead of holding yourself to an unrealistic standard, you can embrace the fact that healthy eating is flexible and can include all kinds of foods that are rich and hearty and delicious, such as pizza. This is a time for you to explore all the options without limiting yourself with old notions of what is good and what is bad. Salad can be very healthy, but it's easy to get fooled into a false sense of health at a salad bar, where options like cheese, meats, and fatty, creamy dressings abound. Sometimes the healthier option *is* the richer option. Learning all you can about food will open your mind to the countless possibilities that won't leave you feeling deprived. You might find that having a guilt-free slice of pizza with your salad is the answer. Mindful eating without deprivation allows you to be an active participant in the ceremony that food plays in the days and events that fill your life.

And since food is a ceremony, why not make it a positive one? Part of the joy of planning your meals is the atmosphere you can create for yourself. Setting a place, sitting down to eat (surprising numbers of people eat standing up!), and savoring each bite all lend to the experience. And be good company for yourself. Whatever you are eating, eat it with purpose and thought. If you feel guilty afterward for what you ate, try not to beat yourself up. Instead, keep a journal about these thoughts, along with good answers that can help you respond to those thoughts the next time you begin beating yourself up over food choices.

This may sound new and foreign, especially if you've never given food or its ceremony much thought. But eating is a ceremony worth focusing on, and can have a profound, lasting impact on how you feel and function.

DIETING SUCCESS

When you have kidney disease and are following the renal diet, you are trying to juggle daily life, your health, and a changing lifestyle. This section will help prepare you for challenges that may arise, and answer some of these questions: "What do I do when I crave something sweet?" and "What do I do when I go out to eat?" I also give you some shopping tips to help you navigate the grocery store like a pro, gravitating toward the good products, and avoiding impulse purchases or unhealthy items.

- **Cravings:** Two things are true of cravings: they're usually short-lived, and there's almost always a substitute. Being prepared is key. If you are prone to cravings, make a list of good distractions (going for a walk, brushing the dog, turning on favorite music, etc.) This way, when cravings arise, you'll have your list to turn to, which can busy your brain long enough for the urge to subside. And keep healthy "craving busters" on hand. If chips and dip are your downfall, would toasted wheat pita or carrots and hummus fill the gap? Maybe some nuts or seeds? If your sweet tooth is the culprit, maybe some sweet berries, baked apples, or frozen yogurt can satisfy that yen. Stock your kitchen wisely, to control what's available to eat!

- **Slipups:** If you give in to an old habit, don't be too hard on yourself. Slipups happen. A temporary lapse does not mean failure, nor does it need to lead to a full-scale relapse. They are called "habits" for a reason—all habits take time to break, just like new ones can take time to develop. In fact, a slipup can provide motivation to try harder, and offer helpful information about what you need to succeed. When you achieve your goals, promise yourself a (nonfood) reward to build your momentum.

- **Shopping:** This is where you can really have some fun. Look at this cookbook for guidance—you can rely on it completely, or use it as a guide. Each weekly meal plan in this book contains a list of all the foods you will need. Check to see if you have the ingredients. Then build your list, integrating those "craving busters" mentioned earlier. Another tip: To avoid impulse buying, go shopping on a full stomach. Research shows that when people are hungry, they're more likely to purchase sweets or other comfort foods that aren't as healthy. Allow yourself enough time in the store to read the nutrition labels. In addition, try to avoid processed foods as much as possible. If it comes in a colorful package, stop and consider: is there a whole foods version of this? For example, that expensive box of flavored rice can be substituted with the real thing, pure and simple, and seasoned by your hand rather than by the manufacturer. You'll use far less salt and avoid the preservatives altogether— and you'll save money!

- **Dining out:** Dining out is a nice treat every once in a while, and there are smart ways to do it. One easy approach to prevent overeating is to share a meal or eat half of your meal at the restaurant, and take the other half home since restaurant portions are often too large anyway. Since we usually go into a restaurant hungry, it's helpful to plan ahead to avoid rash decisions. Most restaurants have their menu available online—check it out for healthy choices that will please you. Try to cut back on fluids and high-potassium foods during the day if you plan to go out for dinner.

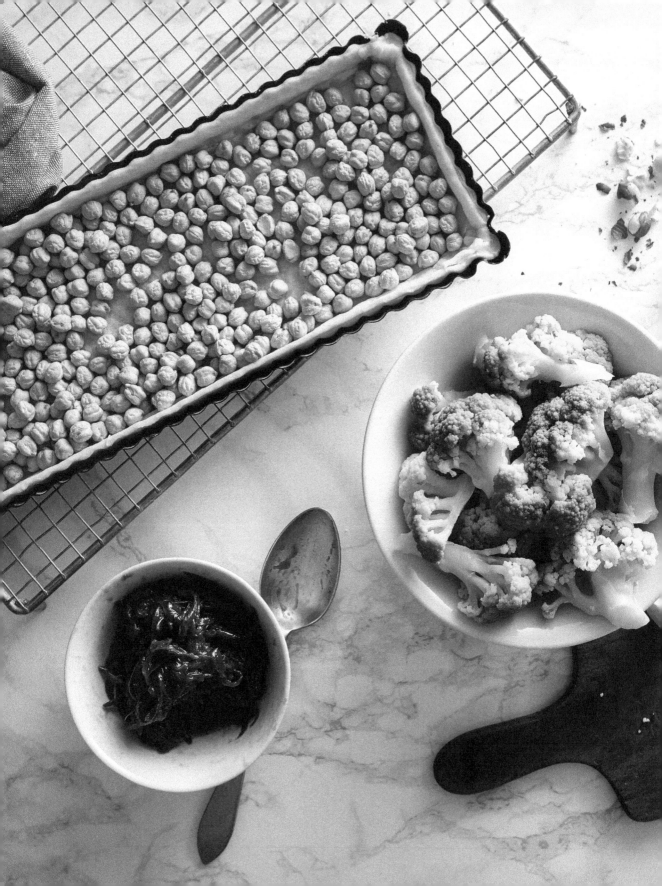

3

THE RENAL DIET
MEAL PLANS

Nobody likes restrictions. And if you're used to cooking a certain way, suddenly being faced with a new list of restrictions can intimidate even the most experienced chef. The goal of this chapter is to give you an idea of what you can eat without worry, while keeping in mind the foods that should be moderated. You'll quickly realize that it is possible to enjoy meals—perhaps more than ever before—regardless of the recommended limitations imposed by renal complications. A basic strategy for sticking with a kidney-healthy diet is to be aware of the nutrient content in your meals and the types of nutrients you may need to limit. For example, you'll be looking to choose the foods with less sodium and the right kinds of protein. This chapter will outline what types of foods to use in everyday meal planning, along with some clever substitutions that will add variety to your plate and help you meet all your nutritional goals.

In this chapter, we'll also look at the dietary rules and principles that should be followed for a successful renal diet. You'll see that while these rules are beneficial for slowing the progression of kidney damage, they are healthy for the general population, as well. So by all means, include your family in your health-supportive menu planning. Lowering sodium intake, for example, will decrease anyone's risk for high blood pressure, while choosing better protein options will decrease saturated fat intake for all diners and, in turn, limit the chances of developing atherosclerosis and heart disease. This chapter will also help you avoid undernutrition by offering a variety of meal options that meet all the important daily needs.

To keep the body functioning properly, we all require essential macronutrients such as fat, carbohydrates, and protein, and micronutrients such as sodium and potassium. Being on the renal diet does not change this fundamental fact. However, it does alter the amounts of certain nutrients that the body can tolerate and process. For example, did you know that 1 teaspoon of table salt equals 2,300 milligrams of sodium? This is already the maximum amount a person should consume in one day! Adjusting for these limitations may seem like a big deal at first, but the information contained in this book will help you change that perception to one of simple awareness about the countless options that exist so you can meet dietary requirements without sacrificing flavor.

As you start on the renal diet, I will be guiding you every step of the way. In the following pages, I have laid out for you three 4-week meal plans—low sodium, low protein, and low fat—with recommended recipes from this book for three meals a day plus a snack. Some general foods you are familiar with are also included in the snacks. I have created each day's meal plan based on the nutrition the meals provide. The recipes in part 2 of this book are all renal-friendly as well as family-friendly. They are easy to prepare, and use affordable, nutritious, easy-to-find ingredients.

THE LOW-SODIUM
RENAL DIET MEAL PLAN

Many of the basic dietary principles on the renal diet are related to fluid. The inability of the kidneys to excrete fluid also means that water-soluble nutrients can build up in the body and cause harmful effects. Certain nutrients, such as sodium, can cause the body to retain fluid, which can increase blood pressure and place added stress on the heart.

There are several ways to limit sodium intake while maintaining a flavorful diet. To control blood pressure, less than 2,300 milligrams of sodium (1 teaspoon) should be consumed per day. This may sound difficult if you're accustomed to keeping a saltshaker on your table, but there are plenty of substitutions that can be made for old-fashioned table salt. For example, substituting dried herbs and seasoning, such as basil and oregano, can maximize flavor without sodium (see Dump the Salt: Explore Your Options, page 46). Keep in mind that there may be sodium hiding in certain store-bought products, so make sure to check the nutrition labels. Also watch out for unwanted sodium in canned or frozen foods. A simple trick is to rinse your canned vegetables or beans prior to eating them, which will eliminate a significant amount of the sodium from the food item. If you buy frozen dinners, look for the low-sodium varieties. But without a doubt, buying fresh, whole foods as often as possible is the best way to control what you are putting in your body.

DUMP THE SALT: EXPLORE YOUR OPTIONS

The science is clear: sodium is of no help to kidneys that are working hard already. But a little experimenting will have you kicking the salt habit as you discover flavorful alternatives that can become your new go-to seasonings. Try some of these tasty, healthier flavor boosters on your meats, grains, and veggies:

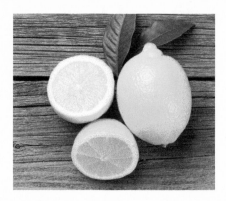

- Beer or wine (use sparingly)
- Cardamom
- Cayenne pepper
- Cilantro
- Cinnamon
- Dill
- Garlic and olive oil (just a small bit of oil will fill your dish with flavor!)
- Lemon
- Rosemary
- Scallions, leeks, onions
- Vinegar (there are countless varieties available)

Don't let the list stop here! The supermarket is packed with great fresh and dried herbs and spices. One caution: Beware of packaged salt substitutes and spice blends that may contain added salt. The best route is always to create your own blend from ingredients you've chosen.

Week 1 Meal Plan

Monday

Breakfast: Blueberry Bread Pudding (page 92)

Lunch: Simple Cabbage Soup (page 121)

Dinner: Marinated Chicken (page 186), Grilled Zucchini and Red Onion Salad (page 139)

Tuesday

Breakfast: Baked Egg Casserole (page 97)

Lunch: Simple Cabbage Soup (leftovers)

Dinner: Stuffed Bell Peppers (page 201)

Wednesday

Breakfast: Blackberry Kale Smoothie (page 81)

Lunch: Cobb Salad (page 143)

Dinner: Pork with Brown Sugar Rub (page 196), Peach Cucumber Salad (page 141)

Thursday

Breakfast: Blueberry Citrus Muffins (page 91)

Lunch: Fish Tacos with Vegetable Slaw (page 176)

Dinner: Vegetable Stew (double recipe, page 128)

Friday

Breakfast: Pretty Pink Smoothie (page 83)

Lunch: Vegetable Stew (leftovers)

Dinner: Homestyle Hamburgers (page 202)

Saturday

Breakfast: Baked Egg Casserole (page 97)

Lunch: Crunchy Chicken Salad Wraps (page 107)

Dinner: Lime Baked Haddock (page 175), Bulgur Vegetable Salad (page 146)

Sunday

Breakfast: Spiced French Toast (page 95)

Lunch: Chicken Alphabet Soup (double recipe, page 124)

Dinner: Ginger Spiced Lamb Chops (page 197), German Braised Cabbage (double recipe, page 111)

Suggested Snacks

Blueberry Citrus Muffins (page 91)

Citrus Sesame Cookies (page 104)

Hardboiled eggs

Grapes

Unsalted popcorn

LOW-
SODIUM
MEAL PLAN

Week 2 Meal Plan

Monday

Breakfast: Apple Pumpkin Muffins (page 90)

Lunch: Chicken Alphabet Soup (leftovers)

Dinner: Baked Cauliflower Rice Cakes (page 159), German Braised Cabbage (leftovers)

Tuesday

Breakfast: Green Kiwi Smoothie (page 84)

Lunch: Citrus Orzo Salad (page 147)

Dinner: Italian Style Meatballs (page 198), Greek Couscous Salad (page 145)

Wednesday

Breakfast: Blueberry Bread Pudding (page 92)

Lunch: Chicken Cabbage Salad (double recipe, page 144)

Dinner: Curried Turkey Bake (page 192)

Thursday

Breakfast: Baked Egg Casserole (page 97)

Lunch: Chicken Cabbage Salad (leftovers)

Dinner: Seared Herbed Scallops (page 170), Herb Roasted Cauliflower (page 109)

Friday

Breakfast: Old-Fashioned Pancakes (page 93)

Lunch: Vibrant Carrot Soup (double recipe, page 120)

Dinner: Pork with Brown Sugar Rub (page 196), Lime Asparagus Spaghetti (page 155)

Saturday

Breakfast: Bell Pepper and Feta Crustless Quiche (page 98)

Lunch: Vibrant Carrot Soup (leftovers)

Dinner: Homestyle Hamburgers (page 202)

Sunday

Breakfast: Tender Oatmeal Pancakes (page 94)

Lunch: Cobb Salad (page 143)

Dinner: Lime Baked Haddock (page 175), Sautéed Butternut Squash (page 110)

Suggested Snacks

Apple Pumpkin Muffins (page 90)

Edamame Guacamole (page 102)

Unsweetened applesauce

Grapes

Vanilla wafer cookies

Week 3 Meal Plan

Monday

Breakfast: Breakfast Tacos (page 96)

Lunch: Peach Cucumber Salad (page 141)

Dinner: Marinated Chicken (page 186), Wild Mushroom Couscous (page 113)

Tuesday

Breakfast: Blackberry Kale Smoothie (page 81)

Lunch: Crunchy Chicken Salad Wraps (page 107)

Dinner: Stuffed Bell Peppers (page 201)

Wednesday

Breakfast: Spiced French Toast (page 95)

Lunch: Citrus Orzo Salad (page 147)

Dinner: Vegetable Stew (double recipe, page 128)

Thursday

Breakfast: Apple Pumpkin Muffins (page 90)

Lunch: Vegetable Stew (leftovers)

Dinner: Italian Style Meatballs (page 198), Walnut Pilaf (page 112)

Friday

Breakfast: Mango Cheesecake Smoothie (page 87)

Lunch: Cobb Salad (double recipe, page 143)

Dinner: Salmon Linguine (page 180)

Saturday

Breakfast: Bell Pepper and Feta Crustless Quiche (page 98)

Lunch: Cobb Salad (leftovers)

Dinner: Pork with Balsamic Vinegar (page 195), Sautéed Butternut Squash (page 110)

Sunday

Breakfast: Tender Oatmeal Pancakes (page 94)

Lunch: Homestyle Chicken Vegetable Stew (page 126)

Dinner: Meatball Soup (double recipe, page 125), Classic Baking Powder Biscuits (page 106)

Suggested Snacks

Apple Pumpkin Muffins (page 90)

Lemon Mousse (page 208)

Watermelon

Vanilla wafer cookies

Carrot sticks

LOW-SODIUM MEAL PLAN

Week 4 Meal Plan

Monday

Breakfast: Old-Fashioned Pancakes (page 93)

Lunch: Meatball Soup (leftovers)

Dinner: Curried Turkey Bake (double recipe, page 192)

Tuesday

Breakfast: Breakfast Tacos (page 96)

Lunch: Curried Turkey Bake (leftovers)

Dinner: Baked Cauliflower Rice Cakes (page 159), Sautéed Butternut Squash (page 110)

Wednesday

Breakfast: Blueberry Bread Pudding (page 92)

Lunch: Chicken Cabbage Salad (page 144)

Dinner: Seared Herbed Scallops (page 170), Zucchini Noodles with Spring Vegetables (page 152)

Thursday

Breakfast: Baked Egg Casserole (page 97)

Lunch: Vibrant Carrot Soup (page 120)

Dinner: Pork with Brown Sugar Rub (page 196), Herb Roasted Cauliflower (page 109)

Friday

Breakfast: Mango Cheesecake Smoothie (page 87)

Lunch: Cobb Salad (page 143)

Dinner: Lentil Veggie Burgers (double recipe, page 158)

Saturday

Breakfast: Spiced French Toast (page 95)

Lunch: Lentil Veggie Burgers (leftovers)

Dinner: Lime Baked Haddock (page 175), Balsamic Pasta Salad (page 134)

Sunday

Breakfast: Bell Pepper and Feta Crustless Quiche (page 98)

Lunch: Crunchy Chicken Salad Wraps (page 107)

Dinner: Homestyle Hamburgers (page 202)

Suggested Snacks

Traditional Spritz Cookies (page 105)

Melon Smoothie Cooler (page 86)

Apple

Rice cakes

Cucumber sticks

THE LOW-PROTEIN
RENAL DIET MEAL PLAN

I n this age of supersized meals, portion control is an important consideration for everyone, but is especially so in the renal diet. Specifically, controlling the amount of protein-rich foods in the diet avoids putting additional stress on the kidneys. However, daily protein requirements still must be met to avoid malnutrition. Animal sources of protein include fish, chicken, meat, eggs, and milk; plant sources include nuts, grains, and beans. It is important to recognize which foods are higher in protein and adjust what you eat based on how much protein you're allowed each day. Some high-protein foods that may need to be eaten in careful moderation include ground beef, chicken breast, tuna, salmon, and shrimp. Lower-protein alternatives include foods like beef stew, egg substitute, and tofu. Beans and grains are another great source of protein, but because of their high protein content, watching how much you eat will be the key to protecting the health of your kidneys. Learn more about which proteins are best for you (see Best Low-Protein Foods, page 29).

Your protein intake may not change significantly in the early stages of CKD. If you are in stages 1, 2, or 3, your protein may be restricted to 12 to 15 percent of your caloric intake each day; the same range recommended by the Dietary Reference Intakes (DRIs) for a healthy diet for normal adults. However, if you're in stage 4, it is recommended that you reduce your protein intake to 10 percent of your caloric intake (see Calculate Your Intake, page 30).

Week 1 Meal Plan

Monday

Breakfast: Green Kiwi Smoothie (page 84)

Lunch: Citrus Orzo Salad (page 147)

Dinner: Cauliflower-Topped Shepherd's Pie (double recipe, page 199)

Tuesday

Breakfast: Blueberry Bread Pudding (page 92)

Lunch: Cauliflower-Topped Shepherd's Pie (leftovers)

Dinner: Sweet Chicken Stir-Fry (page 184)

Wednesday

Breakfast: Baked Vanilla Pudding (page 207)

Lunch: Bean Veggie Tacos (page 150)

Dinner: Shrimp and Greens (page 169), Sautéed Butternut Squash (page 110)

Thursday

Breakfast: Apple Pumpkin Muffins (page 90)

Lunch: Fall Apple Cranberry Salad (page 138)

Dinner: Pork with Brown Sugar Rub (page 196), German Braised Cabbage (page 111)

Friday

Breakfast: Pretty Pink Smoothie (page 83)

Lunch: Lime Asparagus Spaghetti (page 155)

Dinner: Homestyle Chicken Vegetable Stew (double recipe, page 126)

Saturday

Breakfast: Breakfast Tacos (page 96)

Lunch: Homestyle Chicken Vegetable Stew (leftovers)

Dinner: Stuffed Bell Peppers (page 201)

Sunday

Breakfast: Tender Oatmeal Pancakes (page 94)

Lunch: Fish Tacos with Vegetable Slaw (page 176)

Dinner: Sweet Potato Curry (double recipe, page 151)

Suggested Snacks

Apple Pumpkin Muffins (page 90)

Citrus Sesame Cookies (page 104)

Watermelon

Carrot sticks

Graham crackers

Week 2 Meal Plan

Monday

Breakfast: Blackberry Kale Smoothie (page 81)

Lunch: Sweet Potato Curry (leftovers)

Dinner: Sweet Chicken Stir-Fry (page 184)

Tuesday

Breakfast: Old-Fashioned Pancakes (page 93)

Lunch: Simple Cabbage Soup (double recipe, page 121)

Dinner: Salisbury Steak (page 200), Mixed Vegetable Barley (page 163)

Wednesday

Breakfast: Breakfast Tacos (page 96)

Lunch: Simple Cabbage Soup (leftovers)

Dinner: Salmon in Foil Packets (page 177), Bulgur Vegetable Salad (double recipe, page 146)

Thursday

Breakfast: Mango Cheesecake Smoothie (page 87)

Lunch: Bulgur Vegetable Salad (leftovers)

Dinner: Classic Chicken Pot Pie (double recipe, page 188)

Friday

Breakfast: Tender Oatmeal Pancakes (page 94)

Lunch: Classic Chicken Pot Pie (leftovers)

Dinner: Spicy Sesame Tofu with white basmati rice (page 164)

Saturday

Breakfast: Blueberry Bread Pudding (page 92)

Lunch: Balsamic Pasta Salad (page 134)

Dinner: Salmon with Green Vegetables (page 179), Greek Couscous Salad (page 145)

Sunday

Breakfast: Green Kiwi Smoothie (page 84)

Lunch: Fish Tacos with Vegetable Slaw (page 176)

Dinner: Pork with Balsamic Vinegar (page 195), Blueberry Rice Salad (double recipe, page 137)

Suggested Snacks

Edamame Guacamole (page 102)

Toasted Pear Chips (page 103)

Blueberries

Rice cakes

Cauliflower florets

LOW-PROTEIN MEAL PLAN

Week 3 Meal Plan

Monday

Breakfast: Apple Pie Smoothie (page 85)

Lunch: Blueberry Rice Salad (leftovers)

Dinner: Stir-Fried Vegetables with white basmati rice (page 154)

Tuesday

Breakfast: Baked Vanilla Pudding (page 207)

Lunch: Lime Asparagus Spaghetti (page 155)

Dinner: Honey Pork (page 194), Herb Roasted Cauliflower (page 109)

Wednesday

Breakfast: Old-Fashioned Pancakes (page 93)

Lunch: Citrus Orzo Salad (double recipe, page 147)

Dinner: Sweet Chicken Stir-Fry (page 184)

Thursday

Breakfast: Pretty Pink Smoothie (page 83)

Lunch: Citrus Orzo Salad (leftovers)

Dinner: Cauliflower-Topped Shepherd's Pie (double recipe, page 199)

Friday

Breakfast: Breakfast Tacos (page 96)

Lunch: Cauliflower-Topped Shepherd's Pie (leftovers)

Dinner: Salmon in Foil Packets (page 177), Greek Couscous Salad (double recipe, page 145)

Saturday

Breakfast: Tender Oatmeal Pancakes (page 94)

Lunch: Greek Couscous Salad (leftovers)

Dinner: Curried Turkey Bake (double recipe, page 192)

Sunday

Breakfast: Blueberry Bread Pudding (page 92)

Lunch: Curried Turkey Bake (leftovers)

Dinner: Vegetable Stew (double recipe, page 128), Classic Baking Powder Biscuits (page 106)

Suggested Snacks

Traditional Spritz Cookies (page 105)

Spiced Gingerbread (page 212)

Pear

Unsalted popcorn

Popsicles

Week 4 Meal Plan

Monday

Breakfast: Blackberry Kale Smoothie (page 81)

Lunch: Vegetable Stew (leftovers), Classic Baking Powder Biscuits (leftovers)

Dinner: Salisbury Steak (double recipe, page 200), Sautéed Butternut Squash (page 110)

Tuesday

Breakfast: Apple Pumpkin Muffins (page 90)

Lunch: Salisbury Steak (leftovers)

Dinner: Shrimp and Greens (page 169), Mixed Vegetable Barley (page 163)

Wednesday

Breakfast: Mango Cheesecake Smoothie (page 87)

Lunch: Fish Tacos with Vegetable Slaw (page 176)

Dinner: Classic Chicken Pot Pie (double recipe, page 188)

Thursday

Breakfast: Tender Oatmeal Pancakes (page 94)

Lunch: Classic Chicken Pot Pie (leftovers)

Dinner: Pork with Brown Sugar Rub (page 196), Herb Roasted Cauliflower (page 109)

Friday

Breakfast: Baked Vanilla Pudding (page 207)

Lunch: Balsamic Pasta Salad (page 134)

Dinner: Stuffed Bell Peppers (page 201)

Saturday

Breakfast: Breakfast Tacos (page 96)

Lunch: Vibrant Carrot Soup (page 120)

Dinner: Sweet Potato Curry (double recipe, page 151)

Sunday

Breakfast: Old-Fashioned Pancakes (page 93)

Lunch: Sweet Potato Curry (leftovers)

Dinner: Breaded Baked Sole (page 172), Zucchini Noodles with Spring Vegetables (page 152)

Suggested Snacks

Apple Pumpkin Muffins (page 90)

Pretty Pink Smoothie (page 83)

Red bell pepper

Strawberries

Vanilla wafers

LOW-PROTEIN MEAL PLAN

THE LOW-FAT
RENAL DIET MEAL PLAN

Many protein-rich foods are also high in fat, for example red meats and dairy. Choosing low-fat options will help protect your body from the damaging effects of fat accumulation in your blood vessels. This heart-healthy diet is as easy as it gets, because it merely contains a few simple substitutions for a healthier lifestyle. Healthy fats, like those in vegetable oils, can be used as a great source of calories. Simple substitutions like avocado instead of mayonnaise, or olive oil instead of butter, can decrease saturated fat intake while maintaining the rich flavor we all crave. Some adjustments can be made in food preparation as well, which will drastically reduce the amount of saturated fats that end up on your plate. For example, choosing grilled, roasted, or baked options rather than fried reduces fats and protects your heart and kidneys from unnecessary threats. Also, removing the skin from chicken, then adding some bread crumbs and olive oil, can replace the flavor without added fat.

This chapter will provide many options to follow these guidelines while eating a variety of foods. It is possible to reduce sodium and protein, eat heart-healthy meals, and enjoy food more than ever on a renal diet. The next section will give you specific meals to prepare at home, which make the most of the best foods for your dietary needs.

Week 1 Meal Plan

Monday

Breakfast: Blueberry Bread Pudding (page 92)

Lunch: Bean Veggie Tacos (page 150)

Dinner: Crispy Fried Chicken (page 190), Greek Couscous Salad (double recipe, page 145)

Tuesday

Breakfast: Old-Fashioned Pancakes (page 93)

Lunch: Greek Couscous Salad (leftovers)

Dinner: Honey Pork (page 194), Mushroom Rice Noodles (double recipe, page 162)

Wednesday

Breakfast: Raspberry Cucumber Smoothie (page 82)

Lunch: Mushroom Rice Noodles (leftovers)

Dinner: Turkey Barley Stew (double recipe, page 129)

Thursday

Breakfast: Bell Pepper and Feta Crustless Quiche (double recipe, page 98)

Lunch: Turkey Barley Stew (leftovers)

Dinner: Stuffed Bell Peppers (page 201)

Friday

Breakfast: Bell Pepper and Feta Crustless Quiche (leftovers)

Lunch: Zucchini Noodles with Spring Vegetables (page 152)

Dinner: Breaded Baked Sole (page 172), German Braised Cabbage (page 111)

Saturday

Breakfast: Tender Oatmeal Pancakes (page 94)

Lunch: Fish Tacos with Vegetable Slaw (page 176)

Dinner: Steak with Creamy Mustard Sauce (page 203), Bulgur Vegetable Salad (page 146)

Sunday

Breakfast: Breakfast Tacos (page 96)

Lunch: Simple Cabbage Soup (double recipe, page 121)

Dinner: Tunisian Spiced Chicken (page 187), Watermelon Cucumber Salad (page 135)

Suggested Snacks

Papaya Mint Water (page 78)

Baked Vanilla Pudding (page 207)

Raspberries

Unsweetened applesauce

Pear

LOW-FAT MEAL PLAN

Week 2 Meal Plan

Monday

Breakfast: Apple Pie Smoothie (page 85)

Lunch: Simple Cabbage Soup (leftovers)

Dinner: Tangy Orange Shrimp (page 168), Peach Cucumber Salad (page 141)

Tuesday

Breakfast: Blueberry Bread Pudding (page 92)

Lunch: Crunchy Chicken Salad Wraps (page 107)

Dinner: Vegetable Rice Casserole (page 160)

Wednesday

Breakfast: Pretty Pink Smoothie (page 83)

Lunch: Bean Veggie Tacos (page 150)

Dinner: Breaded Baked Sole (page 172), Sautéed Butternut Squash (page 110)

Thursday

Breakfast: Tender Oatmeal Pancakes (page 94)

Lunch: Fish Tacos with Vegetable Slaw (page 176)

Dinner: Stuffed Bell Peppers (page 201)

Friday

Breakfast: Bell Pepper and Feta Crustless Quiche (page 98)

Lunch: Bulgur Vegetable Salad (page 146)

Dinner: Sweet Chicken Stir-Fry (double recipe, page 184)

Saturday

Breakfast: Old-Fashioned Pancakes (page 93)

Lunch: Sweet Chicken Stir-Fry (leftovers)

Dinner: Meatball Soup (double recipe, page 125)

Sunday

Breakfast: Breakfast Tacos (page 96)

Lunch: Meatball Soup (leftovers)

Dinner: Crispy Fried Chicken (page 190), Lime Asparagus Spaghetti (double recipe, page 155)

Suggested Snacks

Melon Smoothie Cooler (page 86)

Toasted Pear Chips (page 103)

Apple

Cucumber sticks

Strawberries

Week 3 Meal Plan

Monday

Breakfast: Raspberry Cucumber Smoothie (page 82)

Lunch: Lime Asparagus Spaghetti (leftovers)

Dinner: Steak with Creamy Mustard Sauce (page 203), Zucchini Noodles with Spring Vegetables (double recipe, page 152)

Tuesday

Breakfast: Blueberry Bread Pudding (page 92)

Lunch: Zucchini Noodles with Spring Vegetables (leftovers)

Dinner: Honey Pork (page 194)

Wednesday

Breakfast: Blackberry Kale Smoothie (page 81)

Lunch: Crunchy Chicken Salad Wraps (page 107)

Dinner: Vegetable Rice Casserole (page 160)

Thursday

Breakfast: Old-Fashioned Pancakes (page 93)

Lunch: Bean Veggie Tacos (page 150)

Dinner: Pesto-Crusted Tilapia (page 174), Lime Asparagus Spaghetti (double recipe, page 155)

Friday

Breakfast: Apple Pie Smoothie (page 85)

Lunch: Lime Asparagus Spaghetti (leftovers)

Dinner: Turkey Barley Stew (page 129)

Saturday

Breakfast: Tender Oatmeal Pancakes (page 94)

Lunch: Fennel Cauliflower Soup (page 122)

Dinner: Crispy Fried Chicken (page 190), Wild Mushroom Couscous (page 113)

Sunday

Breakfast: Bell Pepper and Feta Crustless Quiche (page 98)

Lunch: Fish Tacos with Vegetable Slaw (page 176)

Dinner: Stuffed Bell Peppers (page 201)

Suggested Snacks

Papaya Mint Water (page 78)

Poached Pears (page 206)

Grapes

Celery sticks

Watermelon

LOW-FAT MEAL PLAN

Week 4 Meal Plan

Monday

Breakfast: Pretty Pink Smoothie
(page 83)

Lunch: Bulgur Vegetable Salad
(page 146)

Dinner: Sweet Chicken Stir-Fry
(double recipe, page 184)

Tuesday

Breakfast: Breakfast Tacos (page 96)

Lunch: Sweet Chicken Stir-Fry
(leftovers)

Dinner: Tangy Orange Shrimp
(page 168), Sautéed Butternut
Squash (page 110)

Wednesday

Breakfast: Old-Fashioned Pancakes
(page 93)

Lunch: Simple Cabbage Soup
(double recipe, page 121)

Dinner: Stuffed Bell Peppers
(page 201)

Thursday

Breakfast: Blueberry Bread Pudding
(page 92)

Lunch: Simple Cabbage Soup
(leftovers)

Dinner: Tandoori Chicken (double
recipe, page 191), Sour Cream–
Dressed Cucumbers (double
recipe, page 142)

Friday

Breakfast: Mango Cheesecake
Smoothie (page 87)

Lunch: Tandoori Chicken
(leftovers), Sour Cream–Dressed
Cucumbers (leftovers)

Dinner: Vegetable Rice Casserole
(page 160)

Saturday

Breakfast: Bell Pepper and Feta
Crustless Quiche (page 98)

Lunch: Crunchy Chicken Salad
Wraps (page 107)

Dinner: Steak with Creamy Mustard
Sauce (page 203), Wild Mushroom
Couscous (page 113)

Sunday

Breakfast: Tender Oatmeal
Pancakes (page 94)

Lunch: Bean Veggie Tacos (page 150)

Dinner: Breaded Baked Sole
(page 172), Stir-Fried Vegetables
(page 154)

Suggested Snacks

Melon Smoothie Cooler (page 86)

Toasted Pear Chips (page 103)

Rice cakes

Carrot sticks

PART

2

KIDNEY-FRIENDLY RECIPES

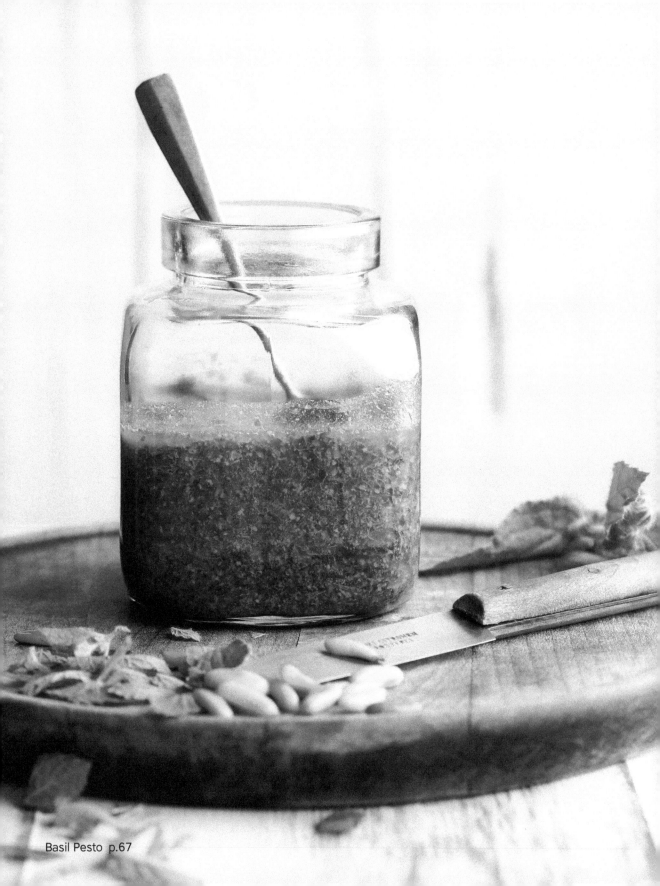

Basil Pesto p.67

4

SEASONINGS, SAUCES, AND CONDIMENTS

SPICY HERB SEASONING

Makes ½ cup / Prep time: 5 minutes

LOW PROTEIN LOW FAT Premade spice and herb seasoning mixes can be a much-appreciated time saver when you want a flavorful meal but don't have the time to create complicated sauces. All you have to do is rub or sprinkle the seasoning mix on your food choice and roast, grill, or broil. This combination of ingredients will work with meats, poultry, seafood, and vegetables, so be sure to have a fresh batch of this handy mixture available at all times.

¼ cup celery seed

1 tablespoon dried basil

1 tablespoon dried oregano

1 tablespoon dried thyme

1 tablespoon onion powder

2 teaspoons garlic powder

1 teaspoon freshly ground black pepper

½ teaspoon ground cloves

1. In a small bowl, stir together the celery seed, basil, oregano, thyme, onion powder, garlic powder, pepper, and cloves.

2. Store in a sealed container in a cool, dark place for up to 1 month.

Substitution tip This spice and herb combination can be altered depending on your taste and spice drawer contents. If you enjoy a hotter blend, add cayenne pepper; if you want a richer flavor, use mild smoked paprika.

PER SERVING (1 teaspoon) Calories: 7; Total fat: 0g; Saturated fat: 0g; Cholesterol: 0mg; Sodium: 2mg; Carbohydrates: 1g; Fiber: 0g; Phosphorus: 9mg; Potassium: 27mg; Protein: 0g

PHOSPHORUS-FREE BAKING POWDER

Makes 1 cup / Prep time: 5 minutes

LOW PROTEIN LOW FAT Baking powder is a staple ingredient in most baking recipes, so why not prepare your own renal diet–friendly version? Regular baking powder contains about 450 mg of phosphorus per teaspoon, which can be too much even in small amounts. The potassium in this recipe is higher than typical baking powder, but is acceptable in small measurements, such as in a baked product.

¾ cup cream of tartar   ¼ cup baking soda

1. In a small bowl, stir together the cream of tartar and baking soda. Sift the mixture together several times to mix thoroughly.

2. Store the baking powder in a sealed container in a cool, dark place for up to 1 month.

Low-sodium tip There are sodium-free and low-sodium versions of baking soda on the market, but they can be hard to find in some areas. You could substitute potassium bicarbonate for the baking soda, but be sure to purchase a product labeled "safe for human consumption."

PER SERVING (1 teaspoon) Calories: 6; Total fat: 0g; Saturated fat: 0g; Cholesterol: 0g; Sodium: 309mg; Carbohydrates: 1g; Fiber: 0g; Phosphorus: 0g; Potassium: 341mg; Protein: 0g

BASIL OIL

Makes 3 cups / Prep time: 10 minutes / Cook time: 4 minutes (plus 2 hours infusing time)

LOW PROTEIN LOW FAT Once you make your first flavored oil and use it in a recipe instead of regular oil, you may become addicted to the art of creating different versions. Basil oil has a sweet flavor that can be drizzled directly on soups and dips, and can be used as a dipping sauce for bread if you want a snack. Try swapping out olive oil for basil oil in salad dressings as well, especially when making Mediterranean-theme recipes.

2 cups olive oil

2½ cups fresh basil leaves, washed and patted dry

1. Place the olive oil and basil leaves in a food processor (or blender), and pulse until the leaves are coarsely chopped.

2. Transfer the mixture to a medium saucepan, and place over medium heat. Heat the oil, stirring occasionally, until it just starts to simmer along the edges, about 4 minutes. Remove from the heat and let it stand until cool, about 2 hours.

3. Pour the oil through a fine-mesh sieve or doubled piece of cheesecloth into a container.

4. Store the basil oil in an airtight glass container in the refrigerator for up to 2 months.

5. Before using for dressings, remove the oil from the refrigerator and let it come to room temperature, or for cooking, scoop out cold spoonfuls.

Substitution tip Flavored oils can be made from any type of herb, not just basil, so have fun experimenting with your favorites. Combinations such as thyme and oregano or chives and dill also work beautifully.

PER SERVING (1 tablespoon) Calories: 40; Total fat: 5g; Saturated fat: 1g; Cholesterol: 0g; Sodium: 0g; Carbohydrates: 0g; Fiber: 0g; Phosphorus: 0g; Potassium: 0g; Protein: 0g

BASIL PESTO

Makes 1½ cups / Prep time: 10 minutes

LOW PROTEIN LOW FAT Pesto is a versatile, delicious condiment made with very few ingredients. Many prepared pestos have unnecessary additives, as well as added salt or sodium-packed seasonings. As is so often the case with prepared foods, making your own pesto is the best method to control exactly what you put in your body. Lemon juice clarifies the taste of the basil here, but for a nice complexity, try balsamic vinegar instead.

2 cups gently packed fresh basil leaves

2 garlic cloves

2 tablespoons pine nuts

¼ cup olive oil

2 tablespoons freshly squeezed lemon juice

1. Put the basil, garlic, and pine nuts in a food processor (or blender), and pulse for about 3 minutes or until very finely chopped.

2. Slowly drizzle the olive oil into the mixture, and pulse until a thick paste forms, scraping down the sides of the bowl at least once.

3. Add the lemon juice, and pulse until well blended.

4. Store the pesto in a sealed glass container in the refrigerator for up to 2 weeks.

Substitution tip Pesto can be made with many herbs, several types of dark leafy greens, and several kinds of nuts, so try out different combinations until you find your favorite mixture.

PER SERVING (1 tablespoon) Calories: 22; Total fat: 2g; Saturated fat: 0g; Cholesterol: 0mg; Sodium: 0mg; Carbohydrates: 0g; Fiber: 0g; Phosphorus: 3mg; Potassium: 10mg; Protein: 0g

SWEET BARBECUE SAUCE

Makes 2 cups / Prep time: 10 minutes / Cook time: 15 minutes

LOW PROTEIN LOW FAT Barbecue sauce has its own culture. There are local and national contests that revolve exclusively around creating the best barbecue sauce recipe—people take consistency and balance of flavors quite seriously. They jealously guard the secret of their sauces and swear by certain ingredients and cooking tricks. This sauce is sweet, slightly salty, and has a subtle bit of heat for a nice balance. Try brushing it on pork, beef, or poultry before grilling or broiling.

1 teaspoon olive oil

½ sweet onion, chopped

1 teaspoon minced garlic

¼ cup honey

¼ cup apple cider vinegar

2 tablespoons low-sodium tomato paste

1 tablespoon Dijon mustard

1 teaspoon hot sauce

1 teaspoon cornstarch

1. Heat the olive oil in a medium saucepan over medium heat.

2. Add the onion and garlic and sauté until softened, about 3 minutes.

3. Stir in ¾ cup water, the honey, vinegar, tomato paste, mustard, and hot sauce.

4. Heat, stirring occasionally, until the mixture is almost simmering, about 6 minutes.

5. In a small cup, stir together ¼ cup of water and the cornstarch.

6. Whisk the cornstarch into the sauce and continue to cook, stirring, until the sauce thickens, about 2 minutes. Cool.

7. Pour the sauce in a sealed glass container and store in the refrigerator for up to 1 week.

Substitution tip Honey adds a touch of sweetness, which enhances the caramelization process of whatever meat or poultry you brush with this sauce. Molasses would also be a lovely substitution for a lusher finish.

PER SERVING (1 tablespoon) Calories: 14; Total fat: 0g; Saturated fat: 0g; Cholesterol: 0g; Sodium: 10mg; Carbohydrates: 3g; Fiber: 0g; Phosphorus: 3mg; Potassium: 17mg; Protein: 0g

LOW-SODIUM MAYONNAISE

Makes 3 cups / Prep time: 15 minutes

LOW PROTEIN Mayonnaise is a delicious simple addition to many dishes, and this healthy version is great to have on hand. Surprisingly, prepared mayonnaise and classic homemade versions contain between 110 mg and 160 mg of sodium per tablespoon, which can be significant when you are watching your diet. This low-sodium recipe allows you to maintain healthy sodium levels in dishes that combine mayonnaise with other ingredients.

2 egg yolks
1 teaspoon Dijon mustard
1 teaspoon honey
2 tablespoons white vinegar

2 tablespoons freshly squeezed lemon
  juice
2 cups olive oil

1. In a large bowl, whisk together the egg yolks, mustard, honey, vinegar, and lemon juice.

2. In a thin stream, whisk in the olive oil until all the oil is used and the mayonnaise is thick and emulsified.

3. Store in a sealed glass container in the refrigerator for up to 2 weeks.

Cooking tip If you want to instantly create the correct texture and consistency, place all the ingredients in a tall glass container and use an immersion blender to mix them. A couple presses of the on/off button to pulse the mixture will whip up perfect mayonnaise with absolutely no effort.

PER SERVING (1 tablespoon) Calories: 83; Total fat: 9g; Saturated fat: 1g; Cholesterol: 9mg; Sodium: 2mg; Carbohydrates: 0g; Fiber: 0g; Phosphorus: 2mg; Potassium: 3mg; Protein: 0g

CITRUS AND MUSTARD MARINADE

Makes ¾ cup / Prep time: 10 minutes

LOW PROTEIN LOW FAT The nutrition numbers listed with this recipe reflect what the ingredients add up to, but they don't necessarily signify what you will be consuming. That number will be significantly lower because you discard most of the marinade after soaking the protein in the bag. Count on about a quarter of the values for a general idea of what you'll be getting in the way of calories, sodium, and other elements.

¼ cup freshly squeezed lemon juice

¼ cup freshly squeezed orange juice

¼ cup Dijon mustard

2 tablespoons honey

2 teaspoons chopped fresh thyme

1. In a medium bowl, whisk together the lemon juice, orange juice, mustard, honey, and thyme until well blended.

2. Store the marinade in a sealed glass container in the refrigerator for up to 3 days. Shake before using.

Substitution tip Any type of citrus fruit works well in this marinade, and all contain the acid required to help tenderize meat, poultry, and fish. Grapefruit, tangerine, lime, and tangelo could all be utilized with great results.

PER SERVING (2 tablespoons) Calories: 35; Total fat: 0g; Saturated fat: 0g; Cholesterol: 0g; Sodium: 118mg; Carbohydrates: 8g; Fiber: 0g; Phosphorus: 14mg; Potassium: 52mg; Protein: 1g

FIERY HONEY VINAIGRETTE

Makes ¾ cup / Prep time: 10 minutes

LOW PROTEIN You might wonder what kind of salad would be enhanced by a "fiery" dressing that packs some heat and a hint of sweetness. Robust-flavored greens like kale and spinach hold their own nicely with this assertive dressing, as do ingredients such as berries, chicken, thin beef slices, tomatoes, and bell peppers. Milder lettuces such as iceberg or Boston might get lost in the dish if you dress them in this commanding vinaigrette. Grilled or broiled shrimp would be delicious drizzled with this sweet heat, as well.

⅓ cup freshly squeezed lime juice

¼ cup honey

¼ cup olive oil

1 teaspoon chopped fresh basil leaves

½ teaspoon red pepper flakes

1. In a medium bowl, whisk together the lime juice, honey, olive oil, basil, and red pepper flakes until well blended.

2. Store the dressing in a sealed glass container in the refrigerator for up to 1 week.

Substitution tip Red pepper flakes are very hot but do not disperse evenly into this dressing, so some bites will pop more than others. If you want to create an even, consistent flavor in your dressing, use ¼ teaspoon of cayenne pepper instead, or even a couple splashes of hot sauce.

PER SERVING (2 tablespoons) Calories: 125; Total fat: 9g; Saturated fat: 1g; Cholesterol: 0mg; Sodium: 1mg; Carbohydrates: 13g; Fiber: 0g; Phosphorus: 1mg; Potassium: 24mg; Protein: 0g

BUTTERMILK HERB DRESSING

Makes 1½ cups / Prep time: 10 minutes

LOW PROTEIN LOW FAT Visions of green farmlands, fields with red barns in the background, and huge, scarred wooden tables heaped with a bounty of homegrown vegetables will dance in your head when you taste this dressing. It's creamy white, tangy, and so very fresh tasting. You might find yourself drizzling it on everything after trying your first bite, and it's pretty low-guilt, so make a double batch to ensure you don't run out.

½ cup skim milk

½ cup Low-Sodium Mayonnaise (page 70)

2 tablespoons apple cider vinegar

½ scallion, green part only, chopped

1 tablespoon chopped fresh dill

1 teaspoon chopped fresh thyme

½ teaspoon minced garlic

Freshly ground black pepper

1. In a medium bowl, whisk together the milk, mayonnaise, and vinegar until smooth.

2. Whisk in the scallion, dill, thyme, and garlic.

3. Season with pepper.

4. Store in a sealed glass container in the refrigerator for up to 1 week.

Ingredient tip The combination of milk and vinegar creates a buttermilk-like flavor without added carbs. You can also use lemon juice or another acid to create the same effect.

PER SERVING (2 tablespoons) Calories: 31; Total fat: 2g; Saturated fat: 0g; Cholesterol: 3mg; Sodium: 19mg; Carbohydrates: 2g; Fiber: 0g; Phosphorus: 13mg; Potassium: 26mg; Protein: 0g

POPPY SEED DRESSING

Makes 2 cups / Prep time: 10 minutes

LOW PROTEIN Many vegetables, fruits, and other salad ingredients are well suited to the renal diet, so having some delicious dressing recipes is almost a must. Poppy seed dressing is a little higher in calories than some others, but is still low in saturated fat, sodium, phosphorus, and potassium—and it's protein-free. These nutrition numbers make it a wonderful choice to reach for during the salad course or a fresh light dinner.

½ cup apple cider or red wine vinegar

⅓ cup honey

¼ cup freshly squeezed lemon juice

1 tablespoon Dijon mustard

1 cup olive oil

½ small sweet onion, minced

2 tablespoons poppy seeds

1. In a small bowl, whisk together the vinegar, honey, lemon juice, and mustard until well blended.

2. Whisk in the oil, onion, and poppy seeds.

3. Store the dressing in a sealed glass container in the refrigerator for up to 2 weeks.

Ingredient tip Culinary poppy seeds are the ripe dried seeds from the same flowers that produce opium. They are highly nutritious, and people are very rarely allergic to them. Other poppy varieties do not produce edible seeds.

PER SERVING (2 tablespoons) Calories: 151; Total fat: 14g; Saturated fat: 2g; Cholesterol: 0mg; Sodium: 12mg; Carbohydrates: 7g; Fiber: 0g; Phosphorus: 13mg; Potassium: 30mg; Protein: 0g

MEDITERRANEAN DRESSING

Makes 1 cup / Prep time: 10 minutes

LOW PROTEIN Cuisine from the Mediterranean area of the world is extremely flavorful and often features oregano as the herbal element in the recipe. Oregano means "delight of the mountain," and has historically been considered the herb of happiness. This fragrant herb is very easy to grow, so try planting some in a garden, window boxes, or a little pot in your kitchen so you can snip a batch for your recipes.

½ cup balsamic vinegar

1 teaspoon honey

½ teaspoon minced garlic

1 tablespoon dried parsley

1 tablespoon dried oregano

½ teaspoon celery seed

Pinch freshly ground black pepper

½ cup olive oil

1. In a small bowl, whisk together the vinegar, honey, garlic, parsley, oregano, celery seed, and pepper.

2. Whisk in the olive oil until emulsified.

3. Store the dressing in a sealed glass container in the refrigerator for up to 1 week.

Substitution tip Fresh herbs can also be used in dressings and sauces. Dried herbs have a more concentrated flavor than fresh, so use about 1 tablespoon of fresh herbs for every teaspoon of dried.

PER SERVING (2 tablespoons) Calories: 100; Total fat: 11g; Saturated fat: 1g; Cholesterol: 0mg; Sodium: 1mg; Carbohydrates: 1g; Fiber: 0g; Phosphorus: 1mg; Potassium: 10mg; Protein: 0g

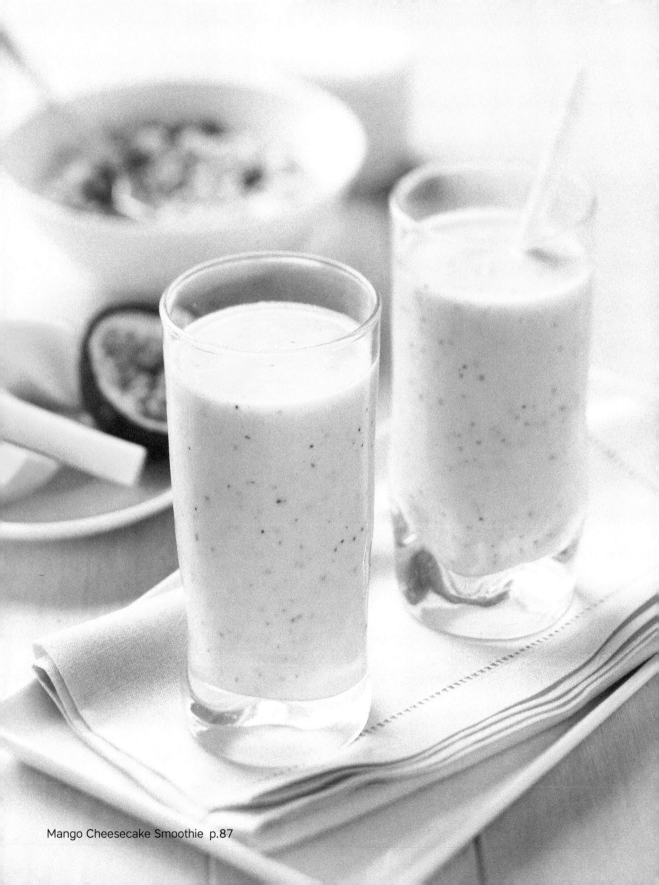

Mango Cheesecake Smoothie p.87

5

SMOOTHIES AND DRINKS

PAPAYA MINT WATER

Serves 10 / Prep time: 5 minutes

LOW PROTEIN LOW FAT Infused water is the trend: it can be found in high-end restaurants, hotel lobbies, and even on college campuses. This refreshing option offers varying benefits, depending on which fruits or herbs are used. You can even purchase special pitchers with fine mesh strainers at the top, so none of the solids come through. If you've never had infused water, you might be surprised at how much flavor actually ends up in your glass. A bonus of making this beverage at home is that the pitcher of bright fruits and herbs looks very pretty sitting in your refrigerator.

1 cup fresh papaya, peeled, seeded, and diced

2 tablespoons chopped fresh mint leaves

10 cups distilled or filtered water

1. Place the papaya and mint in a large pitcher. Pour in the water.
2. Stir, and place the pitcher in the refrigerator to infuse, overnight if possible.
3. Serve cold.

Ingredient tip Papaya comes in many sizes, from fist-size to those that can fill a pitcher by itself. You are simply infusing the water, so any size will work, but a larger fruit will reduce the water volume, and thus, the number of servings it will make.

PER SERVING Calories: 2; Total fat: 0g; Saturated fat: 0g; Cholesterol: 0g; Sodium: 0g; Carbohydrates: 0g; Fiber: 0g; Phosphorus: 0mg; Potassium: 4mg; Protein: 0g

CARROT PEACH WATER

Serves 10 / Prep time: 10 minutes

LOW PROTEIN LOW FAT If you have ever gotten carrot juice on your clothing, the lovely orange color of this infused water will not come as a surprise. This juice is actually an effective fabric and hair dye for those who want to use natural products. In this beverage, the grated carrot very quickly infuses the water in the pitcher with both color and flavor. For a truly glorious hue, pop in a piece of peeled beet as well.

2 peaches, peeled, pitted, and chopped

1 large carrot, peeled and grated

1-inch piece peeled fresh ginger, lightly crushed

3 fresh thyme sprigs

10 cups water

1. Place the peaches, carrot, ginger, and thyme in a large pitcher.

2. Pour in the water, and stir the mixture.

3. Place the pitcher in the refrigerator and leave to infuse, overnight if possible.

4. Serve cold.

Cooking tip Infused water can be replenished when you have emptied the pitcher. Simply leave the fruit, vegetables, and herbs in the bottom, and add more water to infuse overnight again.

PER SERVING Calories: 3; Total fat: 0g; Saturated fat: 0g; Cholesterol: 0g; Sodium: 0g; Carbohydrates: 0g; Fiber: 0g; Phosphorus: 0mg; Potassium: 4mg; Protein: 0g

HOMEMADE RICE MILK

Makes 5 cups / Prep time: 20 minutes

LOW PROTEIN LOW FAT Dairy substitutes are important in the renal diet because one cup of cow's milk has 222 mg of phosphorus and 349 mg of potassium, and goat's milk has even more. Rice milk is a slightly sweet, creamy ingredient that works with most recipes as a dairy milk substitute. You can add a little vanilla extract or other flavoring if you want different options for beverages or meals. Keep some of this milk on hand for the recipes in this book—it can even be frozen. Upon thawing, just stir well to recombine the ingredients.

1 cup cooked white rice

4 cups filtered water, plus more for soaking

1. Put the rice and water in a food processor (or blender), and blend until creamy and smooth, about 4 minutes.

2. Pour the rice milk through a doubled layer of cheesecloth or a fine sieve into a container. Squeeze the rice meal left over in the cloth to remove all the liquid.

3. Discard the rice meal, and store the rice milk in a sealed glass container in the refrigerator for up to 1 week.

Substitution tip Brown rice can be used in this recipe for a nuttier flavor, but this will increase the phosphorus and potassium content in the finished liquid. The amounts are not excessive, but worth being aware of when planning your meals.

PER SERVING (1 cup) Calories: 112; Total fat: 0g; Saturated fat: 0g; Cholesterol: 0mg; Sodium: 80mg; Carbohydrates: 24g; Fiber: 0g; Phosphorus: 0g; Potassium: 55mg; Protein: 0g

BLACKBERRY KALE SMOOTHIE

Serves 2 / Prep time: 5 minutes

LOW PROTEIN LOW FAT Blackberries in their natural state are decadent, plump, and richly hued. They seem to burst with tart juiciness and rich flavor, and so they are perfect for smoothies. If you don't want the seeds in your smoothie, strain them out before putting the liquid back in the blender and adding the ice. Blackberries are packed with vitamin C, fiber, antioxidants, and beneficial phytochemicals.

1 cup fresh or frozen blackberries

½ cup chopped fresh kale, stemmed

1 cup Homemade Rice Milk (page 80; or use unsweetened store-bought)

½ teaspoon vanilla extract

½ teaspoon honey

¼ teaspoon ground cinnamon

3 ice cubes

1. In a blender, put the blackberries, kale, rice milk, vanilla, honey, and cinnamon, and blend until smooth.

2. Add the ice cubes, and blend until thick and smooth.

3. Pour into two tall glasses and serve immediately.

Substitution tip Raspberries and spinach can be substituted for the blackberries and kale for a different tasting smoothie. The color will not be as vibrant, but the finished drink will be sweeter and earthier in flavor.

PER SERVING Calories: 118; Total fat: 1g; Saturated fat: 0g; Cholesterol: 0mg; Sodium: 55mg; Carbohydrates: 25g; Fiber: 4g; Phosphorus: 25mg; Potassium: 193mg; Protein: 2g

RASPBERRY CUCUMBER SMOOTHIE

Serves 2 / Prep time: 5 minutes

LOW PROTEIN LOW FAT Chia seeds are often avoided when kidney disease is an issue, because they are so high in protein. The amount used in this smoothie is not enough to be a concern, and they add more than 50 nutrients, such as fiber, calcium, and omega-3 fatty acids, to the beverage. Chia seeds can absorb about 12 times their weight in liquid, and this helps stabilize blood sugar. Chia seeds can also lower cholesterol, help prevent bone disease, and support weight loss goals.

1 cup fresh or frozen raspberries

½ cup diced English cucumber

1 cup Homemade Rice Milk (page 80; or use unsweetened store-bought) or almond milk

2 teaspoons chia seeds

1 teaspoon honey

3 ice cubes

1. Place the raspberries, cucumber, rice milk, chia seeds, and honey in a blender, and blend until smooth.

2. Add the ice cubes, and blend until thick and smooth.

3. Pour into two tall glasses and serve immediately.

Ingredient tip There are two types of chia seeds, black and white, which have slightly different nutrition profiles. If you are trying to limit your protein, choose the black seeds—they contain less protein.

PER SERVING Calories: 107; Total fat: 1g; Saturated fat: 0g; Cholesterol: 0mg; Sodium: 42mg; Carbohydrates: 25g; Fiber: 1g; Phosphorus: 37mg; Potassium: 135mg; Protein: 5g

PRETTY PINK SMOOTHIE

Serves 2 / Prep time: 5 minutes

LOW PROTEIN LOW FAT Flaxseed add an interesting texture to this smoothie, so if you like a velvety texture, reduce this ingredient to 1 teaspoon instead. Flaxseed are extremely high in omega-3 fatty acids, and are considered the best food source of this important nutrient. Flaxseed promote cardiovascular health, support digestive health, and can help fight cancer and postmenopausal symptoms. Try to incorporate flaxseed regularly in your diet, like with this satisfying smoothie.

½ small cooked beet, peeled and chopped

1 pear, cored and chopped

½ orange, peeled and chopped

1 cup Homemade Rice Milk (page 80; or use unsweetened store-bought)

2 teaspoons flaxseed

1 teaspoon grated peeled fresh ginger

3 ice cubes

1. Place the beet, pear, orange, rice milk, flaxseed, and ginger in a blender, and blend until smooth.

2. Add the ice cubes, and blend until thick and smooth.

3. Pour into two tall glasses and serve immediately.

Ingredient tip Beets come in an assortment of vibrant colors, such as yellow, deep red, and dark purple, which can all create a pretty smoothie. Red beets will make a pastel pink beverage, but the nutrition content is similar in all beets, so experiment with what's fresh and available.

PER SERVING Calories: 137; Total fat: 2g; Saturated fat: 0g; Cholesterol: 0g; Sodium: 50g; Carbohydrates: 29g; Fiber: 4g; Phosphorus: 37mg; Potassium: 197mg; Protein: 1g

GREEN KIWI SMOOTHIE

Serves 2 / Prep time: 5 minutes

LOW PROTEIN LOW FAT The color of this smoothie is decidedly green, unlike some "green" smoothies that are given that name because of their ingredients, despite their sometimes non-green color! Kiwi adds vibrancy to the hue, but it also delivers a hefty nutritional impact. It contains more vitamin C than an orange, ounce for ounce—about 85 percent of the daily recommended amount in one fruit. Kiwi is also high in fiber, helping to regulate blood sugar and support the digestive system.

1 cup water

½ avocado, peeled, pitted, and chopped

1 kiwi, peeled and chopped

½ cup chopped stemmed fresh or
   frozen kale

2 tablespoons almonds

1 teaspoon honey (optional)

2 ice cubes

1. Place the water, avocado, kiwi, kale, almonds, and honey (if using) in a blender, and blend until smooth.

2. Add the ice cubes, and blend until thick and smooth.

3. Pour into two tall glasses and serve immediately.

Cooking tip You'll only be using half an avocado in this recipe, so store the remainder for another recipe or for cutting up over a salad. To avoid discoloration, place the avocado half in a container with some chopped onion, and tightly seal the container.

PER SERVING Calories: 101; Total fat: 6g; Saturated fat: 1g; Cholesterol: 0g; Sodium: 11g; Carbohydrates: 10g; Fiber: 2g; Phosphorus: 63mg; Potassium: 200mg; Protein: 2g

APPLE PIE SMOOTHIE

Serves 2 / Prep time: 5 minutes

LOW PROTEIN LOW FAT You probably would not see spinach in an actual apple pie, unless a creative mother was trying to sneak vegetables into her family's diet. But in this smoothie, the flavorful apples and fragrant warm spices mask the spinach flavor effectively, so you can keep it a secret if you're sharing with a spinach hater. A pinch of nutmeg or ginger would also provide a pleasing contribution if you enjoy a spicy kick.

2 tart apples, cored and chopped

½ cup chopped fresh or frozen spinach

1 cup water

1 teaspoon vanilla extract

½ teaspoon ground cinnamon

Pinch ground cloves

3 ice cubes

1. Place the apples, spinach, water, vanilla, cinnamon, and cloves in a blender, and blend until smooth.

2. Add the ice cubes and blend until thick and smooth.

3. Pour into two tall glasses and serve immediately.

Substitution tip Apples come in a vast variety of types from tart to sweet, but any apple would be delightful in this recipe. Make sure you leave the skin on after scrubbing it so you can benefit from all the fiber and nutrients contained in the skin of this popular fruit.

PER SERVING Calories: 95; Total fat: 0g; Saturated fat: 0g; Cholesterol: 0g; Sodium: 8g; Carbohydrates: 21g; Fiber: 4g; Phosphorus: 20mg; Potassium: 200mg; Protein: 1g

MELON SMOOTHIE COOLER

Serves 2 / Prep time: 5 minutes

LOW PROTEIN LOW FAT If you are used to thick, substantial smoothies, you might find the frothy texture of this drink a fun change. It could almost be poured into a wide cocktail glass and garnished with an umbrella and wedge of fruit. Drink this smoothie quickly, however, because the light texture makes the crushed ice melt quickly. The lemon juice highlights the sweetness of the strawberries and watermelon without adding tartness, so by all means, include it.

1 cup watermelon cubes
½ cup sliced fresh or frozen strawberries
1 tablespoon freshly squeezed lemon juice

1 teaspoon chopped fresh mint leaves
3 ice cubes

1. Place the watermelon, strawberries, lemon juice, and mint in a blender, and blend until smooth.

2. Add the ice cubes, and blend until thick and smooth.

3. Pour into two tall glasses and serve immediately.

Cooking tip When you cut the rind off the watermelon, make sure you leave a little of the pale green section just under the rind attached to the flesh. This often discarded area of the melon is packed with antioxidants, amino acids, and chlorophyll.

PER SERVING Calories: 60; Total fat: 0g; Saturated fat: 0g; Cholesterol: 0g; Sodium: 2g; Carbohydrates: 12g; Fiber: 2g; Phosphorus: 27mg; Potassium: 200mg; Protein: 1g

MANGO CHEESECAKE SMOOTHIE

Serves 2 / Prep time: 5 minutes

LOW PROTEIN LOW FAT The name of this treat conjures visions, doesn't it? It won't disappoint: cream cheese, honey, and sweet mango combine to create a dessert-like drink experience. The milkshake texture can almost be scooped up with a spoon, rather than sipped or sucked through a straw. Garnish the glass with a fresh sprig of mint for an extra-special presentation, or scatter a few fresh berries on top—they will float!

1 cup Homemade Rice Milk (page 80; or use unsweetened store-bought)

½ ripe fresh mango, peeled and chopped

2 tablespoons cream cheese, at room temperature

1 teaspoon honey

½ vanilla bean, split and seeds scraped out

Pinch ground nutmeg

3 ice cubes

1. Place the rice milk, mango, cream cheese, honey, vanilla bean seeds, and nutmeg in a blender, and blend until smooth and thick.

2. Add the ice cubes and blend.

3. Pour into two tall glasses and serve immediately.

Substitution tip If you want to use frozen mango instead of fresh, omit the ice cubes; otherwise the texture will be too thick to suck through a straw.

PER SERVING Calories: 148; Total fat: 1g; Saturated fat: 0g; Cholesterol: 0mg; Sodium: 51mg; Carbohydrates: 36g; Fiber: 4g; Phosphorus: 54mg; Potassium: 133mg; Protein: 2g

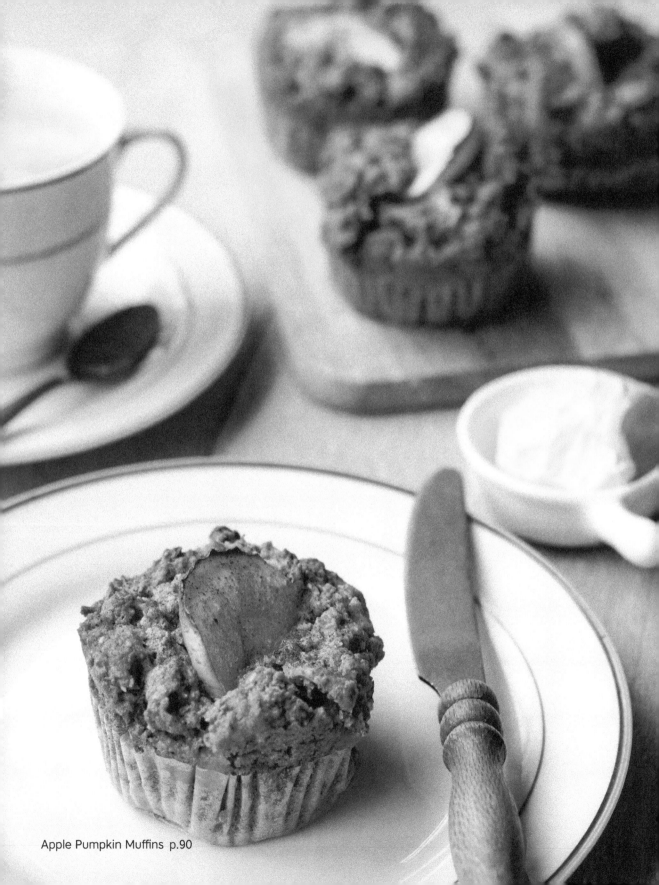

Apple Pumpkin Muffins p.90

6

BREAKFAST

APPLE PUMPKIN MUFFINS

Makes 12 / Prep time: 15 minutes / Cook time: 20 minutes

LOW PROTEIN LOW FAT Bran muffins have a bad reputation with some people because they can be dry and unpalatable if overcooked, and tend to require a generous slathering of butter. You will not need any butter for these muffins, because they are moist with pumpkin and honey. Double up the recipe, because both the batter and the baked muffins freeze beautifully for up to 2 months.

1 cup all-purpose flour

1 cup wheat bran

2 teaspoons Phosphorus Powder (page 65)

1 cup pumpkin purée

¼ cup honey

¼ cup olive oil

1 egg

1 teaspoon vanilla extract

½ cup cored diced apple

1. Preheat the oven to 400°F.

2. Line 12 muffin cups with paper liners.

3. In a medium bowl, stir together the flour, wheat bran, and baking powder.

4. In a small bowl, whisk together the pumpkin, honey, olive oil, egg, and vanilla.

5. Stir the pumpkin mixture into the flour mixture until just combined.

6. Stir in the diced apple.

7. Spoon the batter into the prepared muffin cups.

8. Bake for about 20 minutes, or until a toothpick inserted in the center of a muffin comes out clean.

Ingredient tip Wheat bran is often marketed as just bran, even though there are other types of bran, such as oat, rye, and barley. Bran is simply the hard outer layer of any cereal grain that is stripped away during processing.

PER SERVING (1 muffin) Calories: 125; Total fat: 5g; Saturated fat: 1g; Cholesterol: 18mg; Sodium: 8mg; Carbohydrates: 20g; Fiber: 3g; Phosphorus: 120mg; Potassium: 177mg; Protein: 2g

BLUEBERRY CITRUS MUFFINS

Makes 12 / Prep time: 15 minutes / Cook time: 25 minutes

These muffins are likely to coax even the sleepiest person out of bed! The saturated fat in coconut oil is a medium-chain fatty acid and 50 percent is lauric acid, both of which are easily broken down in the body and have multiple health benefits. Coconut oil can help reduce the risk of diabetes, supports heart health, and fights inflammation in the body.

½ cup coconut oil, melted

1 cup sugar

2 eggs

1 cup Homemade Rice Milk (page 80; or use unsweetened store-bought)

½ cup light sour cream

2 cups all-purpose flour

1 teaspoon freshly grated lemon zest

1 teaspoon freshly grated lime zest

2 teaspoons Phosphorus-Free Baking Powder (page 65)

2 cups fresh blueberries

1. Preheat the oven to 400°F.

2. Line 12 muffin cups with paper liners.

3. In a medium bowl, beat together the coconut oil and sugar with a hand mixer until very fluffy. Then beat in the eggs, rice milk, and sour cream until well blended, scraping down the sides of the bowl.

4. In a small bowl, stir together the flour, lemon zest, lime zest, and baking powder.

5. Stir the flour mixture into the egg mixture until just combined.

6. Stir in the blueberries.

7. Spoon the batter into the prepared muffin cups.

8. Bake about 25 minutes, or until a toothpick inserted in the center of a muffin comes out clean.

Ingredient tip Coconut oil is available in most stores these days because of its upsurge in popularity in the health sector. Look for refined expeller pressed coconut oil, which means it was not extracted using chemicals and is therefore less likely to trigger allergies.

PER SERVING (1 muffin) Calories: 252; Total fat: 9g; Saturated fat: 8g; Cholesterol: 36mg; Sodium: 26mg; Carbohydrates: 38g; Fiber: 1g; Phosphorus: 79mg; Potassium: 107mg; Protein: 4g

BLUEBERRY BREAD PUDDING

Serves 6 / Prep time: 10 minutes (plus 30 minutes soaking time) / Cook time: 35 minutes

LOW FAT Bread pudding has been around for centuries, and is considered an efficient way to use up stale bread. It is also delicious. If you are looking for an impressive meal for guests for brunch or breakfast, assemble the bread pudding the night before, and bake it in the morning while you enjoy your company. No prep work, cleaning up, or slaving in the kitchen—just a seamless presentation.

3 cups Homemade Rice Milk (page 80; or use unsweetened store-bought)

½ cup honey

3 eggs

2 teaspoons vanilla extract

½ teaspoon ground cinnamon

6 cups sourdough bread cubes

2 cups fresh blueberries

1. Preheat the oven to 350°F.

2. In a large bowl, whisk together the rice milk, honey, eggs, vanilla, and cinnamon until well blended.

3. Stir in the bread cubes, and let the mixture soak for 30 minutes.

4. Stir in the blueberries. Spoon the mixture into a 9-by-13-inch baking dish.

5. Bake about 35 minutes, or until a knife inserted in the center comes out clean.

Low-sodium tip Sourdough bread has a delicious tangy flavor but is high in sodium, about 208 mg per slice. Change this ingredient to a low-sodium white bread, and you'll cut the sodium per serving to 156mg.

PER SERVING Calories: 382; Total fat: 4g; Saturated fat: 1g; Cholesterol: 106mg; Sodium: 378mg; Carbohydrates: 67g; Fiber: 3g; Phosphorus: 120mg; Potassium: 170mg; Protein: 11g

OLD-FASHIONED PANCAKES

Serves 4 / Prep time: 15 minutes / Cook time: 12 minutes

LOW PROTEIN LOW FAT Pancakes can be made competently over a shining flat-top in a four-star restaurant or in a battered cast-iron skillet over a banked campfire. All you need is a spatula, a steady hand, and, most importantly, a good recipe. This recipe is as simple as any, except for perhaps the addition of rice milk, which is more kidney-friendly than cow's milk. But you'll enjoy these fluffy golden beauties for a lovely breakfast.

1 cup all-purpose flour

½ cup sugar

½ teaspoon Phosphorus-Free Baking Powder (page 65)

1 cup Homemade Rice Milk (page 80; or use unsweetened store-bought)

2 eggs

1 tablespoon unsalted butter, divided

1. In a medium bowl, stir together the flour, sugar, and baking powder.
2. In a small bowl, whisk together the rice milk and eggs.
3. Add the milk mixture to the flour mixture, and whisk until combined.
4. In a large skillet over medium heat, melt half the butter.
5. Scoop the batter, about ¼ cup for each pancake, into the skillet, and cook the pancakes until the edges are firm and the bottoms are golden, about 3 minutes.
6. Flip the pancakes and cook until golden brown, about 2 minutes.
7. Repeat with the remaining butter and batter.
8. Serve the pancakes hot.

Cooking tip If you have leftover pancakes, let them cool completely and place them in a resealable plastic bag in the refrigerator. When you want to enjoy them, try them cold, or toast them in a toaster.

PER SERVING Calories: 272; Total fat: 6g; Saturated fat: 3g; Cholesterol: 113mg; Sodium: 20mg; Carbohydrates: 49g; Fiber: 1g; Phosphorus: 120mg; Potassium: 131mg; Protein: 6g

TENDER OATMEAL PANCAKES

Serves 4 / Prep time: 15 minutes / Cook time: 12 minutes

LOW PROTEIN LOW FAT Oatmeal adds an interesting toasty flavor to these pancakes that is further enhanced by cooking them in butter. The butter will melt slightly into the cooking pancakes, lightly browning them and creating a luscious nutty taste. Make sure your butter does not get too brown, however, because it can become almost bitter. For a real treat, serve these pancakes with a couple tablespoons of whipped cream.

1 cup all-purpose flour
¼ cup rolled oats
Pinch ground cinnamon

½ cup Homemade Rice Milk (page 80; or use unsweetened store-bought)
1 large egg
1 tablespoon unsalted butter, divided

1. In a medium bowl, stir together the flour, oats, and cinnamon.

2. In a small bowl, whisk together the rice milk and egg.

3. Add the rice milk mixture to the flour mixture, and whisk to combine well.

4. Place a large skillet over medium heat, and melt half the butter.

5. Scoop the batter, about ¼ cup for each pancake, into the skillet, and cook the pancakes until the edges are firm and the bottoms are golden, about 3 minutes.

6. Flip the pancakes and cook until golden brown, about 2 minutes.

7. Repeat with the remaining butter and batter.

8. Serve the pancakes hot.

Ingredient tip Oats come in many different textures, from whole flake products to oats that are cut up finely. The best oats for pancakes are somewhere in the middle, so you don't end up with chunky pancakes or ones that are too heavy.

PER SERVING Calories: 195; Total fat: 5g; Saturated fat: 2g; Cholesterol: 60mg; Sodium: 19mg; Carbohydrates: 30g; Fiber: 2g; Phosphorus: 109mg; Potassium: 92mg; Protein: 6g

SPICED FRENCH TOAST

Serves 4 / Prep time: 15 minutes / Cook time: 12 minutes

The most distinct spice in this dish is cinnamon. This spice is gaining prominence for its positive effect on glucose levels in the body, and has healing properties that come from the essential oils found in cinnamon bark. Cinnamon is also an excellent source of calcium, iron, manganese, and vitamins C, E, and K. Luckily for us, it's delicious too, so what better way to enjoy it than with some delicious French toast?

4 eggs

½ cup Homemade Rice Milk (page 80, or use unsweetened store-bought) or almond milk

¼ cup freshly squeezed orange juice

1 teaspoon ground cinnamon

½ teaspoon ground ginger

Pinch ground cloves

1 tablespoon unsalted butter, divided

8 slices white bread

1. In a large bowl, whisk together the eggs, rice milk, orange juice, cinnamon, ginger, and cloves until well blended.

2. In a large skillet over medium-high heat, melt half the butter.

3. Dredge four of the bread slices in the egg mixture until well soaked, and place them in the skillet.

4. Cook until golden brown on both sides, turning once, about 6 minutes total.

5. Repeat with the remaining butter and bread.

6. Serve 2 pieces of hot French toast to each person.

Cooking tip French toast can easily be made in the oven if you don't want to spend time standing over a skillet. Dredge the bread slices the evening before, and place on a baking sheet in the refrigerator overnight, covered. In the morning, uncover, then pop the pan into a preheated 350°F oven and bake for about 10 minutes, turning once.

PER SERVING Calories: 237; Total fat: 10g; Saturated fat: 4g; Cholesterol: 220mg; Sodium: 84mg; Carbohydrates: 27g; Fiber: 1g; Phosphorus: 119mg; Potassium: 158mg; Protein: 11g

BREAKFAST TACOS

Serves 4 / Prep time: 10 minutes / Cook time: 10 minutes

LOW PROTEIN LOW FAT Time-starved families and busy professionals will appreciate the speed with which this nutritious and attractive breakfast comes together. You'll probably spend more time rinsing out your skillet and putting your coffee cup in the dishwasher than making these tacos. The best part is, you can top this meal with your favorites such as diced avocado, sour cream, or even a sprinkle of cheese if they fit within your diet parameters.

1 teaspoon olive oil

½ sweet onion, chopped

½ red bell pepper, chopped

½ teaspoon minced garlic

4 eggs, beaten

½ teaspoon ground cumin

Pinch red pepper flakes

4 tortillas

¼ cup tomato salsa

1. In a large skillet over medium-high heat, heat the olive oil.

2. Add the onion, bell pepper, and garlic, and sauté until softened, about 5 minutes.

3. Add the eggs, cumin, and red pepper flakes, and scramble the eggs with the vegetables until cooked through and fluffy.

4. Spoon one-fourth of the egg mixture into the center of each tortilla, and top each with 1 tablespoon of salsa.

5. Serve immediately.

Low-sodium tip Most of the sodium in this recipe comes from the tortillas and the prepared salsa—about 287 mg per serving. If you can find low-sodium tortillas and make your own salsa, you can create a breakfast with less than half that amount of sodium per serving.

PER SERVING Calories: 210; Total fat: 6g; Saturated fat: 2g; Cholesterol: 211mg; Sodium: 346mg; Carbohydrates: 17g; Fiber: 1g; Phosphorus: 120mg; Potassium: 141mg; Protein: 9g

BAKED EGG CASSEROLE

Serves 4 / Prep time: 15 minutes / Cook time: 30 minutes

Casseroles aren't just for dinner. They can also serve as a wonderful one-pot solution for brunch or a weekend meal. As with any casserole, you can prepare and assemble the majority of the dish the night before, up to transferring all the cooked vegetables into a baking dish, and cook it the next day after pouring in the eggs.

1 teaspoon olive oil, plus more for the baking dish

½ sweet onion, chopped

½ red bell pepper, chopped

½ teaspoon minced jalapeño pepper

½ teaspoon minced garlic

1 cup chopped fresh spinach

Freshly ground black pepper

8 eggs, beaten

1 tablespoon chopped fresh parsley

1. Preheat the oven to 375°F.
2. Lightly coat an 8-by-8-inch baking dish with olive oil.
3. In a large skillet over medium-high heat, heat 1 teaspoon of olive oil.
4. Sauté the onion, bell pepper, jalapeño pepper, and garlic until softened, about 5 minutes.
5. Add the spinach, and sauté until wilted, about 3 minutes.
6. Season the vegetables with black pepper. Transfer to the prepared baking dish.
7. Pour the eggs over the vegetables, and sprinkle with the parsley.
8. Bake until the eggs are firm, about 20 minutes.
9. Cut into 4 servings and serve.

Cooking tip Leftover casserole is a great cold snack. It can be frozen for up to 2 weeks, cut and wrapped in portions. Remove one from the freezer, microwave for 1 minute, and wrap in a tortilla for a grab-and-go breakfast.

PER SERVING Calories: 128; Total fat: 7g; Saturated fat: 2g; Cholesterol: 282mg; Sodium: 62mg; Carbohydrates: 2g; Fiber: 0g; Phosphorus: 120mg; Potassium: 140mg; Protein: 9g

BELL PEPPER AND FETA CRUSTLESS QUICHE

Serves 5 / Prep time: 15 minutes / Cook time: 25 minutes

LOW FAT Quiche might strike you as a little old-fashioned, maybe a ladies luncheon choice rather than a modern nutritious meal. But quiche is one of the prettiest and most convenient methods of getting a large quantity of nutrients on your plate. Baking the quiche without the crust eliminates calories and fat, and leaves room for a fresh green salad as a crunchy side.

1 teaspoon olive oil, plus more for the pie dish

1 small sweet onion, chopped

1 teaspoon minced garlic

1 red bell pepper, chopped

1 cup Homemade Rice Milk (page 80; or use unsweetened store-bought)

4 eggs

¼ cup all-purpose flour

¼ cup low-sodium feta cheese

2 tablespoons chopped fresh basil leaves

Freshly ground black pepper

1. Preheat the oven to 400°F.

2. Lightly coat a 9-inch pie plate with olive oil.

3. In a medium skillet over medium-high heat, heat 1 teaspoon of olive oil.

4. Add the onion and garlic, and sauté until softened, about 3 minutes.

5. Stir in the bell pepper, and sauté about 3 minutes.

6. Transfer the vegetables to the prepared pie plate.

7. In a medium bowl, whisk together the rice milk, eggs, and flour until blended.

8. Stir in the feta cheese and basil, and season with black pepper.

9. Pour the egg mixture over the vegetables in the pie plate. Bake until the center is set and the edge is golden brown, about 20 minutes.

10. Serve hot, warm, or cold.

PER SERVING Calories: 172; Total fat: 5g; Saturated fat: 3g; Cholesterol: 179mg; Sodium: 154mg; Carbohydrates: 20g; Fiber: 1g; Phosphorus: 120mg; Potassium: 122mg; Protein: 8g

BASIL PORK SAUSAGE

Serves 4 / Prep time: 10 minutes / Cook time: 20 minutes

LOW PROTEIN Sausage is, by definition, seasoned meat, or herbed meat in the case of these basil-enhanced patties. Basil is a world-renowned herb with powerful antibacterial properties and loads of vitamins and minerals including iron, calcium, magnesium, mood-boosting tryptophan, and vitamin A. This fragrant herb can promote a healthy cardiovascular system and reduce the risk or effects of autoimmune diseases such as asthma, rheumatoid arthritis, and inflammatory bowel syndrome.

½ pound ground pork

2 tablespoons chopped fresh basil leaves

1 teaspoon chopped fresh thyme

½ teaspoon chopped fresh sage

¼ teaspoon freshly ground black pepper

1 teaspoon olive oil

1. In a medium bowl, add the pork, basil, thyme, sage, and pepper and mix until well combined.

2. Roll the pork mixture into 12 equal-size balls, then flatten them out.

3. In a large skillet over medium-high heat, heat the olive oil.

4. Fry the pork sausage until cooked through and browned, turning once, about 20 minutes total.

5. Serve hot.

Ingredient tip Ground pork is different from the casing-free sausage meat found in most meat sections of the store, although they are often located side by side. Try to find lean ground pork whenever possible, for a healthier dish.

PER SERVING Calories: 157; Total fat: 13g; Saturated fat: 5g; Cholesterol: 40mg; Sodium: 42mg; Carbohydrates: 0g; Fiber: 0g; Phosphorus: 96mg; Potassium: 161mg; Protein: 9g

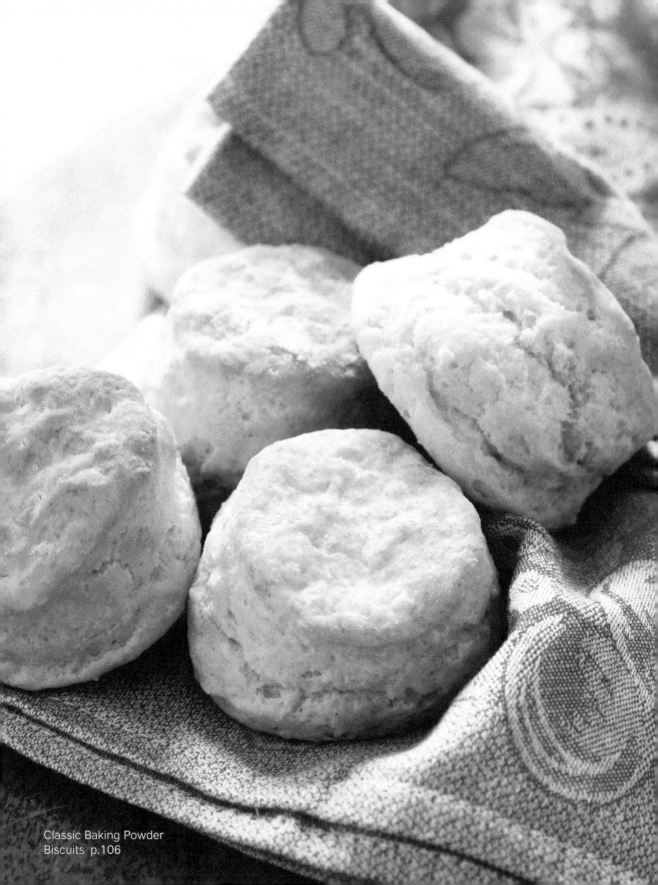

Classic Baking Powder
Biscuits p.106

7

SNACKS AND SIDES

EDAMAME GUACAMOLE

Serves 4 / Prep time: 10 minutes

LOW PROTEIN Guacamole is usually made with avocado, but just a quarter cup of the creamy fruit—the portion size of this recipe—would contain loads (just under 300 mg) of potassium. So, pretty green edamame stands in beautifully for the original. The same portion of edamame is only 140 mg of potassium, more within the guidelines of a kidney-friendly diet. You could add a little avocado to the dish if your diet allows it; just stir the avocado in after puréeing the other ingredients. Serve as a spread or a dip with vegetables, baked pita, or tortilla chips.

1 cup frozen shelled edamame, thawed

¼ cup water

Juice and zest of 1 lemon

2 tablespoons chopped fresh cilantro

1 tablespoon olive oil

1 teaspoon minced garlic

1. In a food processor (or blender), add the edamame, water, lemon juice, lemon zest, cilantro, olive oil, and garlic, and pulse until blended but still a bit chunky.

2. Serve fresh.

Ingredient tip Edamame are young soybeans, before they harden, and can be found shelled or in the pods, both fresh and frozen. For convenience, I recommend using the shelled product.

PER SERVING Calories: 63; Total fat: 5g; Saturated fat: 0g; Cholesterol: 2mg; Sodium: 3mg; Carbohydrates: 1g; Fiber: 0g; Phosphorus: 48mg; Potassium: 152mg; Protein: 3g

TOASTED PEAR CHIPS

Serves 4 / Prep time: 15 minutes / Cook time: 3 to 4 hours

LOW PROTEIN LOW FAT Pears are an elegant fruit, with their graceful curves and delicate skin. But their nutritional content is hearty; pears are packed with fiber, vitamins C and K, as well as copper. Including this pretty fruit as a regular diet choice can help stabilize blood sugar, protect against degenerative diseases, and help prevent cancer. Try a variety—red, green, and pale yellow—for these tempting chips and see which kind becomes your favorite snack.

Olive oil cooking spray

4 firm pears, cored and cut into ⅛-inch-thick slices

2 teaspoons ground cinnamon

1 tablespoon sugar

1. Preheat the oven to 200°F.
2. Line a baking sheet with parchment paper and lightly coat with cooking spray.
3. Spread the pear slices on the baking sheet with no overlap.
4. Sprinkle with the cinnamon and sugar.
5. Bake until the chips are dry, 3 to 4 hours. Cool completely.
6. Store in a sealed container for up to 4 days in a cool, dark place.

Substitution tip If apples are more your style, use 4 small apples instead of pears to make these tasty sweet chips. Peel the apples before slicing them, because the skin can get hard when dried in the oven.

PER SERVING Calories: 101; Total fat: 0g; Saturated fat: 0g; Cholesterol: 0mg; Sodium: 2mg; Carbohydrates: 27g; Fiber: 5g; Phosphorus: 17mg; Potassium: 183mg; Protein: 1g

CITRUS SESAME COOKIES

Makes 18 / Prep time: 15 minutes (plus 1 hour chilling time) / Cook time: 10 minutes

LOW PROTEIN The lush toasty flavor of sesame seeds elevates a basic butter cookie. These seeds are an exceptional source of copper, manganese, iron, and calcium, which together can support respiratory health, prevent vascular disease, help fight cancer, and reduce the severity of premenstrual symptoms.

¾ cup unsalted butter, at room
    temperature

½ cup sugar

1 egg

1 teaspoon vanilla extract

2 cups all-purpose flour

2 tablespoons toasted sesame seeds

½ teaspoon baking soda

1 teaspoon freshly grated lemon zest

1 teaspoon freshly grated orange zest

1. In a large bowl and using a mixer, beat together the butter and sugar on high speed until thick and fluffy, about 3 minutes.

2. Add the egg and vanilla and beat to mix thoroughly, scraping down the sides of the bowl.

3. In a small bowl, stir together the flour, sesame seeds, baking soda, lemon zest, and orange zest.

4. Add the flour mixture to the butter mixture, and stir until well blended.

5. Roll the dough into a long cylinder about 2 inches in diameter, and wrap in plastic wrap. Refrigerate for 1 hour.

6. Preheat the oven to 350°F.

7. Line a baking sheet with parchment paper.

8. Cut the firm cookie dough into ½-inch-thick rounds, and place them on the prepared baking sheet.

9. Bake for 10 to 12 minutes until lightly golden. Cool completely on wire racks.

10. Store in a sealed container in the refrigerator for up to 1 week, or in the freezer for up to 2 months.

PER SERVING (1 cookie) Calories: 150; Total fat: 9g; Saturated fat: 5g; Cholesterol: 32mg; Sodium: 5mg; Carbohydrates: 16g; Fiber: 1g; Phosphorus: 29mg; Potassium: 25mg; Protein: 2g

TRADITIONAL SPRITZ COOKIES

Makes 24 / Prep time: 15 minutes / Cook time: 5 minutes

LOW PROTEIN Spritz cookies have a long history, at least back to the 1500s in Germany. They are named after the German name *Spritzgeback*, which comes from the German verb *spritzen*, meaning to squirt or spray. The cookie press used to create their distinctive shapes basically squirts (or presses) the dough out in patterns. You can use the traditional cookie press for your cookies, but they taste the same—delicious and light—if just scooped out in tablespoons instead.

1 cup unsalted butter, at room
   temperature
½ cup sugar

1 egg
2 teaspoons vanilla extract
2½ cups all-purpose flour

1. Preheat the oven to 400°F.
2. Line a baking sheet with parchment paper.
3. In a large bowl and using a mixer, beat together the butter and sugar on high speed until thick and fluffy, about 3 minutes.
4. Beat in the egg and vanilla, scraping down the sides of the bowl.
5. Beat in the flour on low speed until blended.
6. Drop the cookies by the spoonful onto the prepared baking sheet.
7. Bake until firm and lightly golden, 5 to 7 minutes. Cool completely on a rack.
8. Store in a sealed container in a cool, dry place for up to 1 week.

Cooking tip For a truly authentic spritz cookie, seek out a spritz cookie press at a kitchen store. This device easily creates the signature look of the cookie.

PER SERVING (2 cookies) Calories: 271; Total fat: 16g; Saturated fat: 10g; Cholesterol: 58mg; Sodium: 11mg; Carbohydrates: 26g; Fiber: 1g; Phosphorus: 40mg; Potassium: 39mg; Protein: 3g

CLASSIC BAKING POWDER BISCUITS

Makes 10 biscuits / Prep time: 15 minutes / Cook time: 12 minutes

LOW PROTEIN What could be more comforting than hot steaming biscuits straight out of the oven and nestled in a pretty kitchen cloth–lined basket? You don't really need a basket or a cloth to serve these fluffy golden treats—they might be snatched directly from the baking sheet if you don't supervise your family. Try them with a slather of strawberry jam or a teaspoon of golden honey for a treat, or place a sunny-side-up egg on each half for a more substantial breakfast.

2 cups all-purpose flour

1 tablespoon Phosphorus-Free
   Baking Powder (page 65)

1 tablespoon sugar

½ cup lard

½ cup water

¼ cup Homemade Rice Milk (page 80,
   or use unsweetened store-bought) or
   almond milk

1. Preheat the oven to 350°F.

2. Line a baking sheet with parchment paper.

3. In a large bowl, stir together the flour, baking powder, and sugar.

4. Using your fingertips, rub the lard into the flour mixture until coarse crumbs form. Make a well in the center, and pour in the water and rice milk. Use a fork to toss the mixture until it holds together as a dough. Do not overmix.

5. Pat the dough out on a lightly floured work surface until it is ½ inch thick.

6. Cut out 10 biscuits, and place them on the prepared baking sheet.

7. Bake until light golden brown, 12 to 15 minutes.

Cooking tip For convenience, these biscuits can be frozen, either baked or as dough. Biscuit dough makes a lovely topping for a chicken casserole; just drop pieces of thawed dough on the top of the chicken stew and bake in the oven.

PER SERVING (1 biscuit) Calories: 190; Total fat: 10g; Saturated fat: 4g; Cholesterol: 10mg; Sodium: 45mg; Carbohydrates: 21g; Fiber: 1g; Phosphorus: 27mg; Potassium: 126mg; Protein: 3g

CRUNCHY CHICKEN SALAD WRAPS

Serves 4 / Prep time: 15 minutes

LOW FAT Red grapes provide a pleasing burst of color in this white and green salad, so look for fruit with the deepest red or purple hue. Choosing colorful grapes has a benefit beyond a visual impact: this deep color means the grapes are packed with important flavonoids. The most prevalent is resveratrol, which can cut the risk of cancer, reduce inflammation in the body, and improve blood flow by causing muscle relaxation.

8 ounces cooked shredded chicken

1 scallion, white and green parts, chopped

½ cup halved seedless red grapes

1 celery stalk, chopped

¼ cup Low-Sodium Mayonnaise (page 70) or store-bought mayonnaise

Pinch freshly ground black pepper

4 large lettuce leaves, butter or red leaf

1. In a medium bowl, stir together the chicken, scallion, grapes, celery, and mayonnaise until well mixed.

2. Season the mixture with pepper.

3. Spoon the chicken salad onto the lettuce leaves and serve.

Ingredient tip One of the freshest kinds of butter lettuce you can buy is a hydroponic variety sold with the roots still attached. Most supermarkets carry these heads, and they are so fresh you might swear you could see dew on the leaves.

PER SERVING Calories: 110; Total fat: 3g; Saturated fat: 1g; Cholesterol: 36mg; Sodium: 61mg; Carbohydrates: 6g; Fiber: 0g; Phosphorus: 117mg; Potassium: 200mg; Protein: 13g

TASTY CHICKEN MEATBALLS

Serves 6 / Prep time: 10 minutes / Cook time: 25 minutes

Meatballs are a classic gathering appetizer, often displayed bristled with tooth-picks alongside a tangy dipping sauce. Meatballs are a favorite because they are so easy to make, especially when baked in the oven instead of cooked on the stove, and are the perfect delicious mouthful. This simple base recipe turns out perfectly every time, and the meatballs can be frozen or cooked right away, depending on your needs. Add different herbs or spices to the meat mixture to create your own unique spin.

½ pound lean ground chicken

¼ cup bread crumbs

1 scallion, white and green parts, chopped

1 egg, beaten

1 teaspoon minced garlic

¼ teaspoon freshly ground black pepper

Pinch red pepper flakes

1. Preheat the oven to 400°F.
2. In a large bowl, mix the chicken, bread crumbs, scallion, egg, garlic, black pepper, and red pepper flakes.
3. Form the chicken mixture into 18 meatballs, and place them on a baking sheet.
4. Bake the meatballs for about 25 minutes, turning several times, until golden brown.
5. Serve hot.

Substitution tip Pork, turkey, venison, lamb, and beef can all be used for these meat-balls, as can a combination of several meats. Just swap out the chicken for the same amount of the other ingredient, and proceed as directed.

PER SERVING Calories: 85; Total fat: 4g; Saturated fat: 1g; Cholesterol: 57mg; Sodium: 67mg; Carbohydrates: 4g; Fiber: 0g; Phosphorus: 91mg; Potassium: 200mg; Protein: 8g

HERB ROASTED CAULIFLOWER

Serves 4 / Prep time: 10 minutes / Cook time: 20 minutes

LOW PROTEIN LOW FAT Cauliflower is often smothered in creamy sauces or cheese, so you can't get a real appreciation for the earthy, delicious flavor of the vegetable. Using just fresh herbs and a little olive oil allows that unique taste to shine through, and roasting sweetens the cauliflower a little. If you have leftovers, which is unlikely because it's so good, try adding this tender vegetable to a smoothie or tucking it in a pita with some water-packed tuna as a hearty lunch.

1 tablespoon olive oil, plus more for the pan

1 head cauliflower, cut in half and then into ½-inch-thick slices

1 teaspoon chopped fresh thyme

1 teaspoon chopped fresh chives

¼ teaspoon freshly ground black pepper

1. Preheat the oven to 400°F.

2. Lightly coat a baking sheet with olive oil.

3. Toss the cauliflower, 1 tablespoon of olive oil, the thyme, chives, and pepper until well coated.

4. Spread the cauliflower on the prepared baking sheet.

5. Roast, turning once, until both sides are golden, about 20 minutes.

Ingredient tip Look for cauliflower that is a bright white with no dull or black spots, and has tightly bunched bud clusters. Look for heads surrounded by crisp green leaves to assure the vegetable is freshly picked. If the leaves are limp or dull, the cauliflower is not fresh.

PER SERVING Calories: 82; Total fat: 7g; Saturated fat: 1g; Cholesterol: 0mg; Sodium: 122mg; Carbohydrates: 4g; Fiber: 2g; Phosphorus: 29mg; Potassium: 200mg; Protein: 1g

SAUTÉED BUTTERNUT SQUASH

Serves 8 / Prep time: 10 minutes / Cook time: 20 minutes

LOW PROTEIN LOW FAT Butternut squash is prepared like a vegetable, but is actually classified as a fruit because of its seeds. You might have guessed by the color that this sunny ingredient is very high in beta-carotene, the same antioxidant found in carrots. Butternut squash is also a wonderful source of vitamins A, B_6, C, and E, so it can help reduce the risk of heart disease and boost the immune system. Butternut squash can also help stabilize blood sugar and protect against diabetes and macular degeneration.

1 tablespoon olive oil

4 cups peeled, seeded, 1-inch cubes butternut squash

½ sweet onion, chopped

1 teaspoon chopped fresh thyme

Pinch freshly ground black pepper

1. In a large skillet over medium-high heat, heat the olive oil.

2. Add the butternut squash and sauté until tender, about 15 minutes.

3. Add the onion and thyme, and sauté for 5 minutes.

4. Season with pepper, and serve hot.

Substitution tip Other winter squash are suitable alternatives for this dish if you can't get butternut. Acorn, calabaza, delicata, hubbard, and kabocha are delicious varieties and have a similar nutrition profile to butternut squash.

PER SERVING Calories: 45; Total fat: 1g; Saturated fat: 0g; Cholesterol: 4mg; Sodium: 5mg; Carbohydrates: 7g; Fiber: 1g; Phosphorus: 19mg; Potassium: 200mg; Protein: 1g

GERMAN BRAISED CABBAGE

Serves 4 / Prep time: 15 minutes / Cook time: 15 minutes

LOW PROTEIN LOW FAT The tanginess of German-style braised cabbage comes from the addition of apple cider vinegar. This pale gold vinegar is made from fermented apples and has a complex, slightly sweet flavor that enhances the ingredients of this popular side dish. Apple cider vinegar is a current diet trend because it is thought to have many health benefits. Cider vinegar has long been claimed to help detoxify the body and is a natural diuretic, so it supports kidney health, digestion, and liver function.

1 tablespoon olive oil

5 cups shredded red cabbage

1 pear, peeled, cored, and chopped

¼ large sweet onion, chopped

3 tablespoons apple cider vinegar

1 tablespoon sugar

½ teaspoon caraway seed

½ teaspoon dry mustard

1. In a large skillet over medium-high heat, heat the olive oil.

2. Add the cabbage, pear, and onion, and sauté until tender, about 10 minutes.

3. In a small bowl, stir together the vinegar, sugar, caraway seed, and mustard.

4. Pour the vinegar mixture into the cabbage and stir to combine. Cover and simmer the cabbage for 5 minutes.

5. Serve hot.

Ingredient tip Green cabbage is often the more prevalent variety in supermarkets, so don't despair if you can't find a red one. Green will work fine in this recipe—you just won't get that glorious deep maroon color that looks so inviting on the dinner table.

PER SERVING Calories: 62; Total fat: 2g; Saturated fat: 0g; Cholesterol: 5mg; Sodium: 14mg; Carbohydrates: 10g; Fiber: 3g; Phosphorus: 23mg; Potassium: 161mg; Protein: 1g

WALNUT PILAF

Serves 4 / Prep time: 5 minutes / Cook time: 30 minutes

Roast chicken, spicy grilled pork, and a salsa-topped salmon fillet would all be enhanced by serving this nutty pilaf as an accompaniment. The robust flavor of walnuts needs to be paired with an assertive entrée so it won't overpower the rest of the meal. Whenever possible, try to find black walnuts at the grocery store, because regular walnuts are prone to bitterness and rancidity. Black walnuts are more difficult to find, but have a smooth rich flavor.

1 teaspoon walnut oil

¼ sweet onion, chopped

1 cup white basmati rice

2 cups low-sodium chicken stock

1 tablespoon chopped toasted walnuts

2 tablespoons chopped fresh parsley

1. In a large saucepan over low heat, heat the walnut oil.

2. Add the onion and rice, and sauté for 5 minutes.

3. Stir in the chicken stock, turn the heat to high, and bring the mixture to a boil. Cover, reduce the heat to low, and simmer until the liquid is absorbed, about 25 minutes.

4. Stir in the walnuts and parsley.

5. Serve hot.

Ingredient tip Walnut oil does not stand up to heat well, so don't sauté your ingredients on high. Look for a toasted walnut oil product for a luscious rich flavor in this pilaf.

PER SERVING Calories: 233; Total fat: 5g; Saturated fat: 1g; Cholesterol: 2mg; Sodium: 88mg; Carbohydrates: 41g; Fiber: 1g; Phosphorus: 104mg; Potassium: 179mg; Protein: 6g

WILD MUSHROOM COUSCOUS

Serves 5 / Prep time: 15 minutes / Cook time: 10 minutes

LOW FAT Mushrooms are the only vegetable source of vitamin D, so they can be very important to vegetarians, especially those who live in regions that don't get generous year-round sunlight. Vitamin D has also been shown to help regulate kidney function, which makes this tasty fungus a logical choice for a renal diet. Conversely, don't go overboard with mushrooms, because they are also high in potassium. Moderation is the key.

1 tablespoon olive oil

1 cup mixed wild mushrooms (shiitake, cremini, portobello, oyster, enoki)

¼ sweet onion, finely chopped

1 teaspoon minced garlic

1 tablespoon chopped fresh oregano

3½ cups water

10 ounces couscous

1. In a large skillet over medium-high heat, heat the olive oil.
2. Add the mushrooms, onion, and garlic, and sauté until tender, about 6 minutes.
3. Stir in the oregano and water, and bring the mixture to a boil.
4. Remove the saucepan from the heat, and stir in the couscous.
5. Cover the saucepan and let it stand for 5 minutes.
6. Fluff the couscous with a fork, and serve.

Ingredient tip For a dramatic presentation, try to source Israeli couscous, which is quite a bit larger than regular couscous. Israeli couscous takes a little longer to absorb the water or liquid, so factor in extra time if you are using this product.

PER SERVING Calories: 237; Total fat: 3g; Saturated fat: 0g; Cholesterol: 6mg; Sodium: 7mg; Carbohydrates: 44g; Fiber: 3g; Phosphorus: 115mg; Potassium: 165mg; Protein: 8g

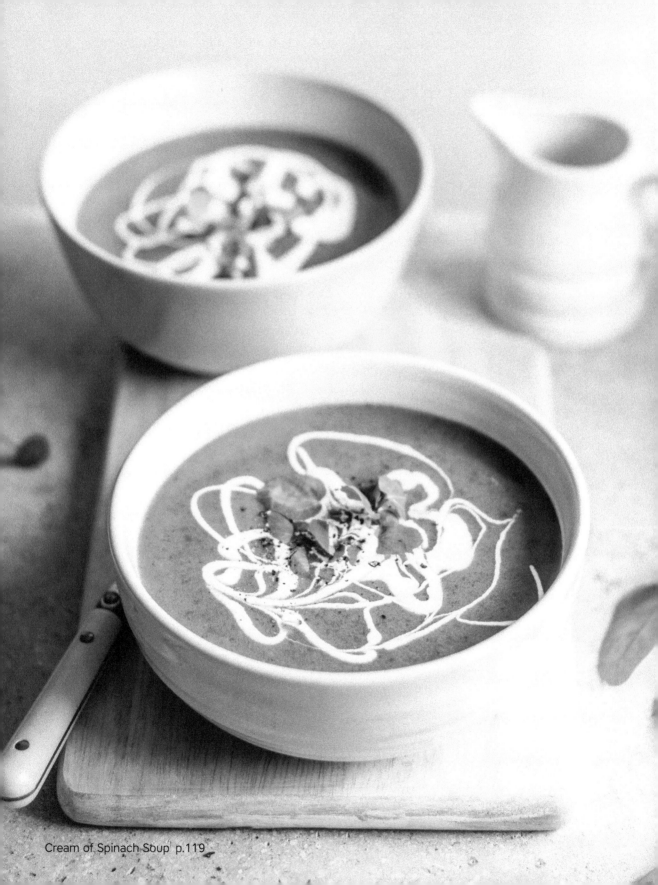

Cream of Spinach Soup p.119

8

SOUPS AND STEWS

EASY LOW-SODIUM CHICKEN BROTH

Makes 8 cups / Prep time: 10 minutes / Cook time: 4 hours

LOW PROTEIN LOW FAT Homemade chicken stock might seem like a great deal of effort when there are good prepared products available, but there is a real satisfaction and value in producing an ingredient that you control. Chicken stock does not need to have preservatives, lots of sodium, or ingredients that don't add flavor to the mix. Stock can be stored for two months in the freezer, so whenever you have the ingredients and time, whip up a batch for your recipes.

2 pounds skinless whole chicken, cut into pieces

4 garlic cloves, lightly crushed

2 celery stalks, with greens, roughly chopped

2 carrots, roughly chopped

1 sweet onion, cut into quarters

10 peppercorns

4 fresh thyme sprigs

2 bay leaves

Water

1. In a large stockpot, place the chicken, garlic, celery, carrots, onion, peppercorns, thyme, and and bay leaves, and cover with water by about 3 inches.

2. Bring the water to a boil over high heat, then reduce the heat to medium-low and simmer, uncovered, for about 4 hours.

3. Skim off any foam on top of the stock, and pour the stock through a fine-mesh sieve.

4. Pick off all the usable chicken meat for another recipe, discard the bones and other solids, and allow the stock to cool for about 30 minutes before transferring it to sealable containers.

5. Store the stock in the refrigerator for up to 1 week, or in the freezer for up to 2 months.

Ingredient tip If you enjoy making roast chicken for dinner, keep the carcasses after you have stripped off all the meat, and store the bones in a resealable bag in the freezer. Once you have two or three bags saved, you can use the carcasses to make this stock.

PER SERVING (1 cup) Calories: 32; Total fat: 0g; Saturated fat: 0g; Cholesterol: 0g; Sodium: 57mg; Carbohydrates: 8g; Fiber: 0g; Phosphorus: 50mg; Potassium: 187mg; Protein: 1g

PESTO GREEN VEGETABLE SOUP

Serves 6 / Prep time: 10 minutes / Cook time: 15 minutes

LOW PROTEIN Think of verdant meadows and you might get close to the lavish green of this fresh-tasting soup. The snow peas in the recipe seem to have a flavor you can drink in, so juicy and new. Summer is the best time of year to serve this soup that features so much ripe, in-season produce, so visit your local farmers' market for fresh ingredients and invite some special guests to share this meal.

2 teaspoons olive oil

1 leek, white and light green parts, sliced
   and washed thoroughly

2 celery stalks, diced

1 teaspoon minced garlic

2 cups sodium-free chicken stock

1 cup chopped snow peas

1 cup shredded spinach

1 tablespoon chopped fresh thyme

Juice and zest of ½ lemon

¼ teaspoon freshly ground black pepper

1 tablespoon Basil Pesto (page 67)

1. In a large saucepan over medium-high heat, heat the olive oil.

2. Add the leek, celery, and garlic, and sauté until tender, about 3 minutes.

3. Stir in the stock, and bring to a boil.

4. Stir in the snow peas, spinach, and thyme, and simmer for about 5 minutes.

5. Remove the pan from the heat, and stir in the lemon juice, lemon zest, pepper, and pesto.

6. Serve immediately.

Low-sodium tip Commercially prepared pesto has about 145 mg of sodium per tablespoon. Making your own pesto from fresh basil leaves, olive oil, fresh garlic, and freshly ground black pepper allows you to decrease that sodium amount per tablespoon down to zero.

PER SERVING Calories: 170; Total fat: 13g; Saturated fat: 3g; Cholesterol: 2g; Sodium: 333mg; Carbohydrates: 8g; Fiber: 1g; Phosphorus: 42mg; Potassium: 200mg; Protein: 3g

VEGETABLE MINESTRONE

Serves 6 / Prep time: 20 minutes / Cook time: 20 minutes

LOW PROTEIN LOW FAT Minestrone is a substantial soup with a long history in Italy, often made from whatever vegetables are in season at the time. This version does not contain the traditional pasta or beans, but still serves as a robust meal when you crave something warm and filling after a long day. You can add some kidney beans or noodles if you wish; just stir them in with the stock, and simmer until cooked through and tender.

1 teaspoon olive oil

½ sweet onion, chopped

1 celery stalk, diced

1 teaspoon minced garlic

2 cups sodium-free chicken stock

2 medium tomatoes, chopped

1 zucchini, diced

½ cup shredded stemmed kale

Freshly ground black pepper

1 ounce grated Parmesan cheese

1. In a large saucepan over medium-high heat, heat the olive oil.

2. Add the onion, celery, and garlic, and sauté until softened, about 5 minutes.

3. Stir in the stock, tomatoes, and zucchini, and bring to a boil.

4. Reduce the heat to low, and simmer for 15 minutes.

5. Stir in the kale, and season with pepper.

6. Garnish with the Parmesan cheese, and serve.

Low-sodium tip There is not much sodium in this recipe, but you could cut it further by omitting the Parmesan cheese. One tablespoon of Parmesan has about 80 mg of sodium.

PER SERVING Calories: 100; Total fat: 3g; Saturated fat: 1g; Cholesterol: 7mg; Sodium: 195mg; Carbohydrates: 6g; Fiber: 1g; Phosphorus: 70mg; Potassium: 200mg; Protein: 4g

CREAM OF SPINACH SOUP

Serves 4 / Prep time: 15 minutes / Cook time: 30 minutes

LOW PROTEIN Spinach might not be your first choice for a soup base—it feels more like a salad or side dish—but this leafy dark green has an assertive flavor that holds its own in a soup. The lemon juice brightens the green's taste even more. For a memorable presentation, drizzle the heavy cream over the finished soup rather than blending it in.

1 tablespoon olive oil

½ sweet onion, chopped

2 teaspoons minced garlic

4 cups fresh spinach

¼ cup chopped fresh parsley

3 cups water

¼ cup heavy (whipping) cream

1 tablespoon freshly squeezed lemon juice

Freshly ground black pepper

1. In a large saucepan over medium-high heat, heat the olive oil.

2. Add the onion and garlic, and sauté until soft, about 3 minutes.

3. Add the spinach and parsley, and sauté for 5 minutes.

4. Stir in the water, bring to a boil, then reduce the heat to low. Simmer the soup until the vegetables are tender, about 20 minutes.

5. Cool the soup for about 5 minutes, then, along with the heavy cream, purée the soup in batches in a food processor (or a blender, or with a handheld immersion blender).

6. Return the soup to the pot, and warm through on low heat.

7. Add the lemon juice, season with pepper, and stir to combine.

8. Serve hot.

Substitution tip Any dark leafy green can be used in place of spinach for this elegant soup. Kale, watercress, Swiss chard, and even beet greens all combine well with the other ingredients, and have a similar nutrition profile to spinach.

PER SERVING Calories: 141; Total fat: 14g; Saturated fat: 7g; Cholesterol: 48mg; Sodium: 36mg; Carbohydrates: 3g; Fiber: 1g; Phosphorus: 38mg; Potassium: 200mg; Protein: 2g

VIBRANT CARROT SOUP

Serves 4 / Prep time: 15 minutes / Cook time: 25 minutes

LOW PROTEIN The carrot isn't the only star in this colorful soup. The turmeric has a distinctive flavor often included in curries and Asian cuisine. Beyond its kitchen applications, in many cultures this pungent spice is used medicinally as an anti-inflammatory and antioxidant. These properties are important for reducing the risk of kidney infections and preventing inflammation in the body. Turmeric also contains curcumin, a plant chemical that is being studied for its potential anti-cancer effect.

1 tablespoon olive oil

½ sweet onion, chopped

2 teaspoons grated peeled fresh ginger

1 teaspoon minced fresh garlic

4 cups water

3 carrots, chopped

1 teaspoon ground turmeric

½ cup coconut milk

1 tablespoon chopped fresh cilantro

1. In a large saucepan over medium-high heat, heat the olive oil.

2. Sauté the onion, ginger, and garlic until softened, about 3 minutes.

3. Stir in the water, carrots, and turmeric. Bring the soup to a boil, reduce the heat to low, and simmer until the carrots are tender, about 20 minutes.

4. Transfer the soup in batches to a food processor (or blender), and process with the coconut milk until the soup is smooth. Return the soup to the pan and reheat.

5. Serve topped with the cilantro.

Ingredient tip The turmeric in this recipe adds the technicolor brightness to the soup, not the carrots. Turmeric has been a popular fabric dye in many cultures for thousands of years.

PER SERVING Calories: 113; Total fat: 10g; Saturated fat: 6g; Cholesterol: 0mg; Sodium: 30mg; Carbohydrates: 7g; Fiber: 2g; Phosphorus: 50mg; Potassium: 200mg; Protein: 1g

SIMPLE CABBAGE SOUP

Serves 8 / Prep time: 20 minutes / Cook time: 35 minutes

LOW PROTEIN LOW FAT Cabbage is the main ingredient in this hearty soup and a wonderful choice for any diet because it is inexpensive and very nutritious. Cabbage is a cruciferous vegetable—one of the vegetables recommended to eat every day, like broccoli, Brussels sprouts, cauliflower—and packed with phytochemicals that fight inflammation caused by free radicals in the body. Cabbage is also low in potassium, and is a good source of fiber, vitamins C and K, and folic acid.

1 tablespoon olive oil

½ sweet onion, chopped

2 teaspoons minced garlic

6 cups water

1 cup sodium-free chicken stock

½ head green cabbage, shredded

2 carrots, diced

2 medium tomatoes, diced

Freshly ground black pepper

2 tablespoons chopped fresh thyme

1. In a large saucepan over medium-high heat, heat the olive oil.

2. Add the onion and garlic, and sauté until softened, about 3 minutes.

3. Stir in the water, chicken stock, cabbage, carrots, and tomatoes, and bring to a boil. Reduce the heat to medium-low and simmer until the vegetables are tender, about 30 minutes.

4. Season the soup with black pepper. Serve hot, topped with the thyme.

Cooking tip To save time, you can purchase a package of coleslaw mix instead of shredding your own cabbage and carrots. Since this recipe only uses half a cabbage head, buying premade might reduce food waste.

PER SERVING Calories: 62; Total fat: 2g; Saturated fat: 0g; Cholesterol: 1mg; Sodium: 61mg; Carbohydrates: 6g; Fiber: 2g; Phosphorus: 32mg; Potassium: 200mg; Protein: 2g

FENNEL CAULIFLOWER SOUP

Serves 6 / Prep time: 20 minutes / Cook time: 30 minutes

LOW FAT Fennel is an underutilized vegetable in most North American households, partly because most home cooks do not know what to do with it and partly because the licorice taste is unusual and unfamiliar. If you examine the delicate fronds that top this vegetable and eat a small raw piece, you might detect that fennel is in the same family as dill, carrots, and parsley. Fennel is a stellar source of fiber, which can help control blood sugar and reduce cholesterol.

2 C chicken Broth

1 teaspoon olive oil

1 small sweet onion, chopped

2 teaspoons minced garlic

½ small head cauliflower, cut into small florets

2 cups chopped fresh fennel

4 cups water, or as much as needed to cover the vegetables

2 teaspoons chopped fresh thyme

¼ cup heavy (whipping) cream

1. In a large saucepan over medium-high heat, heat the olive oil.

2. Add the onion and garlic, and sauté until softened, about 3 minutes.

3. Add the cauliflower, fennel, and water. Bring to a boil, then reduce the heat to medium-low and simmer until the cauliflower is tender, about 20 minutes.

4. In batches, pour the soup into a food processor (or blender), and purée until smooth and creamy.

5. Return the soup to the pan, and stir in the thyme and cream. Heat on medium-low until warmed through, about 5 minutes.

6. Serve.

Cooking tip This soup freezes well, so double the recipe to create some leftovers for a convenient meal another day. Just omit the heavy whipping cream from the leftover portion, and add it when you reheat the soup.

PER SERVING Calories: 105; Total fat: 8g; Saturated fat: 5g; Cholesterol: 27mg; Sodium: 30mg; Carbohydrates: 5g; Fiber: 2g; Phosphorus: 41mg; Potassium: 200mg; Protein: 1g

MUSHROOM MOCK MISO SOUP

Serves 6/ Prep time: 35 minutes / Cook time: 10 minutes

LOW PROTEIN LOW FAT The spare ingredients in this clear soup allow the fresh ginger to shine through and infuse each spoonful. Ginger has been used for thousands of years as an important remedy for many ailments, touted mostly for its anti-inflammatory and antioxidant benefits; you may have taken it for stomach upset in the form of ginger ale. This spice also supports the kidneys; it helps the kidneys move toxins through more effectively, helping rid them from the body.

6 cups water, divided

2 ounces dried mixed mushrooms

¼ cup seasoned rice vinegar

1 teaspoon low-sodium soy sauce

1 tablespoon grated peeled fresh ginger

1 cup julienned snow peas

½ cup grated carrot

2 scallions, green and white parts, chopped

1. Put 2 cups of water in a small saucepan over high heat, and bring to a boil. Place the dried mushrooms in a medium bowl, and pour the boiling water over them. Let the mushrooms reconstitute for 30 minutes, then remove them from the water and slice them thinly.

2. Transfer the mushroom water, the remaining 4 cups of water, vinegar, soy sauce, and ginger to a large saucepan, and place over medium-high heat. Bring to a boil, and add the mushrooms, snow peas, and carrot. Reduce the heat to low, and simmer for 5 minutes.

3. Serve hot, topped with the scallions.

Ingredient tip The ingredient combination in this recipe gives a close approximation to miso, without the intensity of flavor. Real miso contains too much sodium to be effective on a renal diet —about 1,100 mg per ounce!

PER SERVING Calories: 56; Total fat: 0g; Saturated fat: 0g; Cholesterol: 0g; Sodium: 118mg; Carbohydrates: 9g; Fiber: 9g; Phosphorus: 43mg; Potassium: 198mg; Protein: 2g

CHICKEN ALPHABET SOUP

Serves 6 / Prep time: 15 minutes / Cook time: 35 minutes

LOW FAT When you were a child and were sick at home in bed, you might remember that there was nothing better than a steaming bowl of homemade chicken soup to soothe your throat and spirits. Adorable noodles shaped like letters create a whimsical effect that is just fun and, as a bonus, delicious. You can replace the alphabet noodles with more traditional noodles, but let's admit it, even adults can appreciate a meal that you can spell words with while you eat.

1 tablespoon olive oil

½ sweet onion, diced

2 teaspoons minced garlic

4 cups water

1½ cups chopped cooked chicken breast

1 cup sodium-free chicken stock

2 celery stalks, chopped

1 carrot, peeled and diced

½ cup dried alphabet noodles

Freshly ground black pepper

2 tablespoons chopped fresh parsley

1. In a large saucepan over medium-high heat, heat the olive oil.

2. Add the onion and garlic, and sauté until softened, about 3 minutes.

3. Add the water, chicken, chicken stock, celery, and carrot. Bring to a boil, then reduce the heat to medium-low and simmer until the vegetables are tender-crisp, about 15 minutes.

4. Add the noodles, stir, and simmer the soup until the noodles are tender, about 15 minutes.

5. Season with pepper and serve hot, topped with the parsley.

Ingredient tip You may never have noticed the small box of alphabet noodles in the pasta section of your supermarket unless you were looking for it. Select regular noodles rather than whole-wheat to keep the phosphorus and potassium levels lower.

PER SERVING Calories: 132; Total fat: 3g; Saturated fat: 1g; Cholesterol: 36mg; Sodium: 95mg; Carbohydrates: 10g; Fiber: 1g; Phosphorus: 116mg; Potassium: 200mg; Protein: 13g

MEATBALL SOUP

Serves 6 / Prep time: 20 minutes / Cook time: 40 minutes

LOW FAT Watch out! This recipe might become a new family favorite. The broth that results from cooking the raw meatballs right in it, and the addition of fresh celery greens, make for a hearty and satisfying dish. Celery greens are often thrown away because home cooks don't realize these leafy center stalks are a valuable ingredient. In fact, celery greens are high in fiber, calcium, vitamin E, and iodine, which means they boost the immune system, support the nervous system, and can help protect your body from free radicals.

½ pound lean ground beef

2 tablespoons bread crumbs

1 tablespoon chopped fresh parsley

1 teaspoon minced garlic

1 teaspoon olive oil

½ sweet onion, chopped

5 cups water

2 tomatoes, chopped

2 celery stalks with the greens, chopped

1 carrot, diced

Freshly ground black pepper

1. In a large bowl, mix together the ground beef, bread crumbs, parsley, and garlic, and roll the meat mixture into small (1-inch) meatballs.

2. In a large saucepan over medium-high heat, heat the olive oil. Add the onion, and sauté until softened, about 3 minutes.

3. Add the water, tomatoes, celery, and carrot, and bring to a boil. Add the meatballs, reduce the heat to medium-low, and simmer until the vegetables are tender and the meatballs are cooked through, about 35 minutes.

4. Season the soup with pepper, and serve hot.

Cooking tip Add the raw meatballs to the simmering soup in this recipe, because as the meat cooks in the broth, it imparts a rich, beefy taste to the liquid. Since you are using water as the base instead of stock or broth, this flavor transfer is crucial for the final soup.

PER SERVING Calories: 106; Total fat: 3g; Saturated fat: 1g; Cholesterol: 23mg; Sodium: 53mg; Carbohydrates: 4g; Fiber: 1g; Phosphorus: 92mg; Potassium: 200mg; Protein: 9g

HOMESTYLE CHICKEN VEGETABLE STEW

Serves 6 / Prep time: 20 minutes / Cook time: 50 minutes

LOW PROTEIN Chunks of bright carrot are popular in stews because they can stand up to long hours of braising or simmering. And this root vegetable also contains beta-carotene, which can reduce the risk of hypertension, a prevailing issue in CKD. But carrots are high in potassium, so enjoy them within the parameters of your individual dietary needs.

1 teaspoon olive oil

½ pound boneless, skinless chicken breast, cut into 1-inch cubes

½ sweet onion, chopped

1 tablespoon minced garlic

2 cups water

1 cup sodium-free chicken stock

2 celery stalks, sliced

1 sweet potato, peeled and sliced

1 carrot, sliced

1 cup cauliflower florets

1 tablespoon chopped fresh thyme

2 tablespoons water

2 teaspoons cornstarch

¼ cup heavy (whipping) cream

Freshly ground black pepper

1. In a large saucepan over medium-high heat, heat the olive oil. Add the chicken, and sauté until lightly browned, stirring often, about 6 minutes.

2. Add the onion and garlic, and sauté until softened, about 3 minutes.

3. Add the water, chicken stock, celery, sweet potato, and carrot, and bring the stew to a boil. Reduce the heat to medium-low, and simmer until the chicken is cooked through and tender, about 30 minutes.

4. Add the cauliflower and thyme, and simmer 5 more minutes.

5. In a small bowl, stir together the water and cornstarch, and add the mixture to the stew. Stir to incorporate the cornstarch mixture, and simmer until the stew thickens, 3 to 4 minutes.

6. Remove from the heat, and season with pepper before serving.

Cooking tip Yams and sweet potatoes are often confused and the names used interchangeably, but they are not the same vegetable. Avoid yams in this recipe because they have over 800 mg more potassium per cup than do sweet potatoes.

PER SERVING Calories: 101; Total fat: 5g; Saturated fat: 2g; Cholesterol: 25mg; Sodium: 31mg; Carbohydrates: 9g; Fiber: 3g; Phosphorus: 81mg; Potassium: 200mg; Protein: 5g

VEGETABLE STEW

Serves 8 / Prep time: 15 minutes / Cook time: 15 minutes

LOW PROTEIN LOW FAT Onion might seem like just another flavoring in this abundant vegetable dish, but it is actually a powerful tool to help you reach your health goals. Onion is low in potassium and very high in flavonoids—natural chemicals that support the cardiovascular system and nervous system as well as detoxify the body. Onions are particularly high in the antioxidant flavonoid quercetin. Flavonoids are most concentrated in the outer layers of the onion, so take off just the papery layers of peel and leave as much flesh as possible.

1 teaspoon olive oil

1 sweet onion, chopped

1 teaspoon minced garlic

2 zucchini, chopped

1 red bell pepper, diced

2 carrots, chopped

2 cups low-sodium vegetable stock

2 large tomatoes, chopped

2 cups broccoli florets

1 teaspoon ground coriander

½ teaspoon ground cumin

Pinch cayenne pepper

Freshly ground black pepper

2 tablespoons chopped fresh cilantro

1. In a large saucepan over medium-high heat, heat the olive oil. Add the onion and garlic, and sauté until softened, about 3 minutes.

2. Add the zucchini, bell pepper, and carrots, and sauté for 5 minutes.

3. Stir in the vegetable stock, tomatoes, broccoli, coriander, cumin, and cayenne pepper. Bring to a boil, then reduce the heat to medium-low and simmer until the vegetables are tender, stirring often, about 5 minutes.

4. Season with pepper and serve hot, topped with the cilantro.

Low-sodium tip All commercial stocks and broths have added sodium, even the ones labeled "low sodium." Your best strategy to control this mineral is to make your own stocks. Vegetable stock is the easiest because it's just water and an assortment of vegetables and herbs of your choosing, simmered for about 1 hour on low. After simmering, just strain and use! Or store in the freezer in airtight containers for up to 2 months.

PER SERVING Calories: 45; Total fat: 1g; Saturated fat: 0g; Cholesterol: 0g; Sodium: 194mg; Carbohydrates: 5g; Fiber: 1g; Phosphorus: 21mg; Potassium: 184mg; Protein: 1g

TURKEY BARLEY STEW

Serves 6 / Prep time: 25 minutes / Cook time: 45 minutes

LOW FAT Turkey stew or soup is usually a spin-off from a huge festive holiday meal when you have lots of turkey meat left over. This stew uses raw turkey, so you can enjoy it whenever the fancy strikes you or you see turkey breasts on sale at the supermarket. Cooking the turkey breast from raw, in chunks, ensures that the meat is juicy and doesn't fall apart when you simmer the rest of the ingredients. The flavor of the meat also infuses nicely into the cooking broth.

1 teaspoon olive oil

½ pound uncooked turkey breast, cut into ½-inch pieces

½ sweet onion, chopped

1 teaspoon minced garlic

3 cups water

1 cup sodium-free chicken stock

1 cup shredded green cabbage

1 carrot, sliced

½ cup barley

2 bay leaves

2 tablespoons fresh parsley leaves

Freshly ground black pepper

1. In a large saucepan over medium-high heat, heat the olive oil. Add the turkey, and sauté until cooked through, about 7 minutes.

2. Add the onion and garlic, and sauté until softened, about 3 minutes.

3. Add the water, stock, cabbage, carrot, barley, and bay leaves. Bring to a boil, then reduce the heat to low, and simmer until the barley and vegetables are tender, about 35 minutes.

4. Remove the bay leaves, and stir in the parsley.

5. Season with pepper, and serve hot.

Ingredient tip You might not think there is any real difference in onions, but in the renal diet, the type of onion you use is important. Sweet onions have less potassium, about 40 mg per onion, than regular cooking onions.

PER SERVING Calories: 117; Total fat: 1g; Saturated fat: 0g; Cholesterol: 23mg; Sodium: 29mg; Carbohydrates: 15g; Fiber: 3g; Phosphorus: 118mg; Potassium: 200mg; Protein: 11g

BRAISED BEEF MUSHROOM STEW

Serves 6 / Prep time: 15 minutes / Cook time: 1 hour and 10 minutes

Besides the aromatics, garlic and onion, the predominant flavoring in this dish is fresh thyme. Thyme has a distinctive, clean taste and is a popular addition in Mediterranean and French foods, where it's often combined with basil and oregano in recipes. Thyme is a good source of iron, calcium, magnesium, and vitamins A, C, and E. The herb is also very high in flavonoids and can help boost immunity and detoxify the body.

2 tablespoons olive oil

½ pound beef chuck roast, trimmed of fat, cut into 1-inch chunks

½ sweet onion, chopped

2 teaspoons minced garlic

½ cup red wine

1 cup water, plus 2 tablespoons

2 cups halved mushrooms, woody ends trimmed

1 teaspoon chopped fresh thyme

1 teaspoon cornstarch

Freshly ground black pepper

1 tablespoon chopped fresh parsley, for garnish

1. Preheat the oven to 400°F.

2. In a large skillet over medium-high heat, heat the olive oil. Add the beef chunks, and sauté until lightly browned on all sides, about 5 minutes. Remove the beef with a slotted spoon and set aside on a plate.

3. Add the onion and garlic to the skillet, and sauté for 3 minutes.

4. Stir in the red wine and deglaze the skillet, using a wooden spoon to scrape up any flavorful browned bits on the bottom of the pan.

5. Transfer the vegetables and liquid and drippings from the skillet to a large covered casserole dish.

6. Add 1 cup of water, the beef and any drippings on the plate, and the mushrooms and thyme.

7. Cover the casserole dish tightly with a lid or foil, and place in the oven. Braise the stew until the meat is very tender, stirring occasionally, about 1 hour. Put on the stove top over medium heat.

8. In a small bowl, stir together the remaining 2 tablespoons of water and the cornstarch, then stir the mixture into the hot stew to thicken the sauce.

9. Season the stew with pepper, and serve hot, topped with the parsley.

Cooking tip Stew can be made easily and conveniently in a slow cooker if you have this handy appliance in your kitchen. Cook the stew on low heat for 9 hours or on high for 6 hours.

PER SERVING Calories: 146; Total fat: 8g; Saturated fat: 2g; Cholesterol: 24mg; Sodium: 22mg; Carbohydrates: 2g; Fiber: 0g; Phosphorus: 99mg; Potassium: 199mg; Protein: 9g

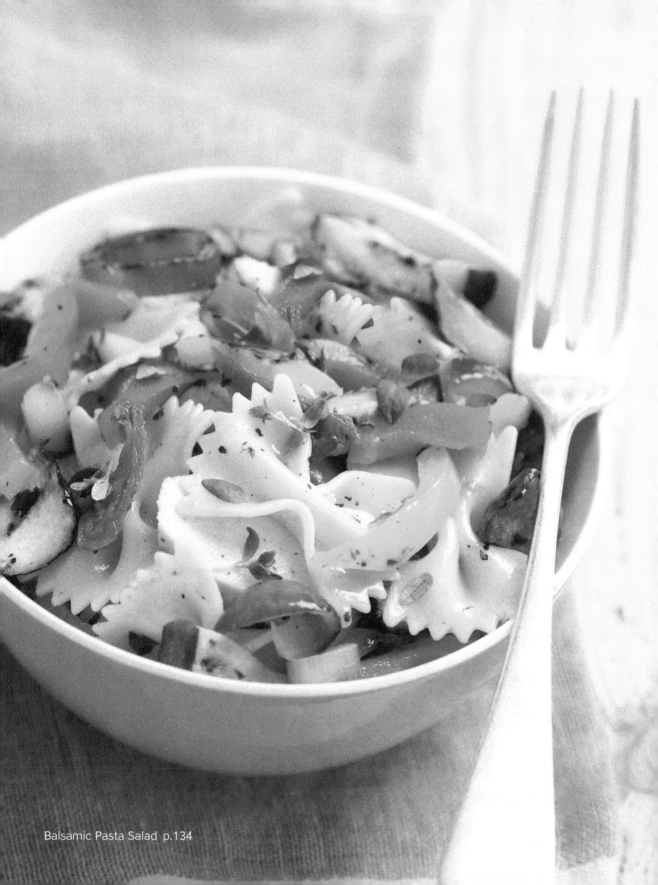

Balsamic Pasta Salad p.134

9

SALADS

BALSAMIC PASTA SALAD

Serves 4 / Prep time: 15 minutes / Cook time: 5 minutes

LOW PROTEIN Pasta salad is a vibrant side dish, but also stands in nicely as a main course. You can use any type of pasta, but these frilled bowties add a fun element. Make this salad the day before so the flavors can mellow and deepen.

3 tablespoons olive oil, divided

2 tablespoons balsamic vinegar

½ scallion, white and green parts, chopped

Freshly ground black pepper

1 zucchini, cut lengthwise into ¼-inch-wide strips

1 red bell pepper, cut in half lengthwise and seeded

1 yellow bell pepper, cut in half lengthwise and seeded

½ red onion, cut into ¼-inch disks

3 cups cooked farfalle pasta

1. Preheat the oven to broil.

2. Line a baking sheet with aluminum foil.

3. In a small bowl, whisk together 2 tablespoons of olive oil, the vinegar, and scallion, and season with pepper.

4. In a large bowl, add the zucchini, red bell pepper, yellow bell pepper, and onion, and toss with the remaining 1 tablespoon of olive oil.

5. Spread the vegetables on the prepared baking sheet. Broil, flipping once, until softened and lightly charred, about 3 minutes total.

6. Dice the zucchini, cut the bell peppers into strips, and chop the onion.

7. Put the vegetables back in the large bowl, add the farfalle and the dressing, and toss to coat. Serve.

Ingredient tip Real balsamic vinegar can be hard to come by in many places, except in Italy, where it is strictly regulated and aged a minimum of 12 years. If you are paying five dollars an ounce or less for your balsamic vinegar in the US, it is most likely just white vinegar with grape juice. But don't let that stop you—this dish still tastes great either way.

PER SERVING Calories: 303; Total fat: 12g; Saturated fat: 3g; Cholesterol: 50mg; Sodium: 12mg; Carbohydrates: 41g; Fiber: 1g; Phosphorus: 111mg; Potassium: 150mg; Protein: 5g

WATERMELON CUCUMBER SALAD

Serves 6 / Prep time: 20 minutes

LOW PROTEIN LOW FAT Watermelon seems to be the defining food for summer picnics and lazy days spent on the dock. It is impossible to eat wedges of watermelon neatly because it is so juicy, which is what makes it such an excellent kidney-friendly food. Watermelon helps the body produce more urine because it is a natural diuretic. This means more waste products leave the body and your kidneys are healthier.

3 cups diced watermelon

1 English cucumber, diced

1 cup halved cherry tomatoes

1 scallion, white and green parts, chopped

2 tablespoons freshly squeezed lemon juice

1 tablespoon chopped fresh cilantro

1. In a large bowl, add the watermelon, cucumber, tomatoes, scallion, lemon juice, and cilantro, and toss together to mix.

2. Chill the salad in the refrigerator for 30 minutes before serving.

Cooking tip If you chop the ingredients in this salad more finely, you can create a gorgeous salsa to serve with fish or with baked unsalted tortilla chips. Throw in a minced jalapeño pepper for a bit of heat.

PER SERVING Calories: 42; Total fat: 0g; Saturated fat: 0g; Cholesterol: 0mg; Sodium: 3mg; Carbohydrates: 9g; Fiber: 1g; Phosphorus: 27mg; Potassium: 200mg; Protein: 1g

BLUEBERRY RICE SALAD

Serves 4 / Prep time: 15 minutes

LOW PROTEIN You might think you are looking at artwork when this glorious salad is scooped onto your plate. A multitude of colors and textures makes this a lovely first course or side dish with almost any meal. Mint adds to the pleasing melange of flavors—its cool taste comes from the compound menthol. Mint helps stimulate digestion and cleanses the blood. This popular herb is also an excellent source of calcium, manganese, iron, and vitamins A and C.

1 cup cooked white basmati rice

1 scallion, white and green parts, chopped

1 red bell pepper, chopped

½ cup shredded carrot

½ cup shredded stemmed kale

1 cup fresh blueberries

2 tablespoons freshly squeezed lemon juice

2 tablespoons chopped fresh mint leaves

1 tablespoon olive oil

Freshly ground black pepper

1. In a large bowl, add the rice, scallion, bell pepper, carrot, kale, and blueberries. Toss together gently.

2. In a small bowl, whisk together the lemon juice, mint, and olive oil and season with pepper.

3. Add the dressing to the salad, and toss to combine.

4. Serve.

Substitution tip Barley, bulgur, or couscous could stand in nicely if you want something a little more exotic than plain white rice. You can even mix several cooked grains together to create texture and an interesting taste experience.

PER SERVING Calories: 176; Total fat: 5g; Saturated fat: 1g; Cholesterol: 0mg; Sodium: 20mg; Carbohydrates: 31g; Fiber: 4g; Phosphorus: 101mg; Potassium: 200mg; Protein: 3g

BERRY SUMMER SALAD

Serves 4 / Prep time: 15 minutes

LOW PROTEIN LOW FAT Many salads are so coated in dressing that you can't even taste the individual ingredients at all. Conversely, this salad has no dressing, but you will not miss it because the sweet berries are perfect when combined with just a hint of basil. All the berries featured here are nutritious, but blueberries are considered a superfood because they are packed with disease-fighting antioxidants. They're also low on the glycemic index, can help lower cholesterol, and are high in fiber, which can help stabilize blood sugar.

4 cups shredded red leaf lettuce

1 cup sliced fresh strawberries

1 cup fresh raspberries

1 cup fresh blueberries

1 tomato, diced

2 tablespoons chopped pistachio nuts

2 tablespoons chopped fresh basil leaves

1. Divide the lettuce, berries, and tomato among four plates.

2. Top each salad with equal amounts of pistachios and basil.

3. Serve.

Substitution tip Although the mixture of three different berries produces a beautiful salad, you can use a single variety if the others aren't available or are too expensive.

PER SERVING Calories: 82; Total fat: 3g; Saturated fat: 1g; Cholesterol: 6mg; Sodium: 87mg; Carbohydrates: 13g; Fiber: 4g; Phosphorus: 63mg; Potassium: 200mg; Protein: 3g

FALL APPLE CRANBERRY SALAD

Serves 5 / Prep time: 20 minutes

LOW PROTEIN Cranberries are a popular home remedy for preventing urinary tract infections because they can help stop bacteria growth in the bladder and kidneys. Cranberries are high in fiber, vitamin C, and antioxidants, and low in natural sugar, which is why they are so tart. Cranberries are not in season year-round, so frozen products and reduced-sugar sauces are sometimes the only options at the grocery store for this superfood. Cranberries freeze really well, so when they are in season and stocked in the stores, grab some for your freezer.

FOR THE DRESSING

3 tablespoons olive oil

2 tablespoons apple cider vinegar

2 tablespoons cranberry sauce
  (see Ingredient tip)

1 teaspoon Dijon mustard

½ teaspoon chopped thyme

FOR THE SALAD

2 cups shredded spinach

2 cups finely shredded cabbage

2 apples, cored and diced

¼ cup chopped walnuts

1 scallion, white and green parts,
  chopped

TO MAKE THE DRESSING

In a small bowl, whisk together the olive oil, vinegar, cranberry sauce, mustard, and thyme. Set aside.

TO MAKE THE SALAD

1. In a large bowl, toss together the spinach, cabbage, apples, walnuts, and scallion.

2. Add the dressing, toss to coat, and serve.

Ingredient tip Cranberries are plump, rosy red, and mouth-puckeringly tart. This tartness is the reason most cranberry sauces are packed with added sugar. If you want to limit your sugar consumption, you can make your own cranberry sauce—it only takes about 5 minutes! Simmer whole berries in a little water and a bit of sugar until they pop and the mixture thickens (use only half or less of the suggested water and sugar in the package recipe).

PER SERVING Calories: 159; Total fat: 12g; Saturated fat: 2g; Cholesterol: 0mg; Sodium: 18mg; Carbohydrates: 13g; Fiber: 3g; Phosphorus: 43mg; Potassium: 198mg; Protein: 2g

GRILLED ZUCCHINI AND RED ONION SALAD

Serves 4 / Prep time: 15 minutes / Cook time: 10 minutes

LOW PROTEIN Olive oil is a key component of the dressing in this recipe and is also an important ingredient for general good health because it is anti-inflammatory. Olive oil is typically linked to supporting the cardiovascular system, but it's also very good for the kidneys. It is a monounsaturated fat; one of the properties of this fat is its ability to protect against oxidative stress, which has been implicated in renal disease.

6 zucchini, both green and yellow, cut into ¼-inch-thick slices

½ medium red onion, thinly sliced

¼ cup olive oil

Freshly ground black pepper

3 tablespoons balsamic vinegar

2 tablespoons chopped fresh oregano

1. Preheat a barbecue grill to medium heat.

2. In a medium bowl, toss the zucchini and onion with the olive oil, and season with pepper.

3. Grill the zucchini and onion until lightly charred, turning once, about 4 minutes per side.

4. Transfer the grilled vegetables to a large bowl, and let them cool for about 30 minutes.

5. Toss the grilled vegetables with the balsamic vinegar and the oregano, and serve.

Cooking tip If you do not have a barbecue, you can broil the vegetables until they are tender and lightly charred, turning once, about 4 minutes per side. They won't have that distinctive barbecue flavor, but the salad will still be a treat.

PER SERVING Calories: 140; Total fat: 14g; Saturated fat: 2g; Cholesterol: 0g; Sodium: 4g; Carbohydrates: 4g; Fiber: 0g; Phosphorus: 23mg; Potassium: 115mg; Protein: 1g

WALNUT ASPARAGUS RIBBON SALAD

Serves 4 / Prep time: minutes

LOW PROTEIN Garlic is not a subtle flavoring and it packs a strong nutritional punch along with its assertive flavor. The garlic in this salad's dressing is not overwhelming, but rather a fleeting taste on the tongue. Its power here is anti-inflammatory: garlic is linked to preventing several diseases and improving many conditions. It can kill bacteria that can damage the kidneys, while protecting these organs against inflammation. Since garlic works best when consumed raw, this salad is a perfect meal choice.

FOR THE DRESSING
2 tablespoons olive oil
1 tablespoon rice vinegar
1 tablespoon honey
1 teaspoon grated peeled fresh ginger
½ teaspoon chili paste
½ teaspoon minced garlic
Juice and zest of 1 fresh lemon

FOR THE SALAD
15 asparagus spears, trimmed, stalks cut into thin ribbons with a peeler
1 cup shredded stemmed kale
2 tablespoons chopped fresh mint leaves
¼ cup chopped walnuts

TO MAKE THE DRESSING
In a small bowl, whisk together the oil, vinegar, honey, ginger, chili paste, garlic, lemon juice, and lemon zest. Set aside.

TO MAKE THE SALAD
1. In a large bowl, toss together the asparagus, kale, mint, and walnuts.
2. Add the dressing, toss until the ingredients are well coated, and serve.

Cooking tip If you chop, slice, and dice lots of vegetables, you might want to consider buying a mandoline. This tool has parallel and horizontal blades that can create mounds of cut vegetables, and can also make fabulous crosshatch patterns in firm vegetables.

PER SERVING Calories: 129; Total fat: 12g; Saturated fat: 1g; Cholesterol: 0mg; Sodium: 9mg; Carbohydrates: 5g; Fiber: 2g; Phosphorus: 61mg; Potassium: 199mg; Protein: 3g

PEACH CUCUMBER SALAD

Serves 4 / Prep time: 15 minutes

LOW PROTEIN LOW FAT If you've ever visited a farmers' market in the summer, you may have experienced the scent of ripe peaches in a stall before you actually saw the rosy fruit. Peaches are one of the most luscious fruits, and their sweetness is perfect mixed with fresh cucumber in this salad. Peaches are high in vitamin C, fiber, and beta-carotene. They promote healthy skin and eyes, detoxify the body, and support the digestive system.

1 peach, peeled, pitted, and diced into ½-inch cubes

1 English cucumber, diced into ½-inch cubes

½ cup halved cherry tomatoes

1 scallion, white and green parts, chopped

½ cup chopped fresh mint leaves

1 tablespoon freshly squeezed lime juice

4 cups mixed baby greens

Freshly ground black pepper

1. In a large bowl, toss together the peach, cucumber, tomatoes, scallion, mint, and lime juice.

2. Arrange the greens on four plates, and top with the peach mixture.

3. Season the salad with pepper, and serve.

Ingredient tip When choosing peaches for recipes such as this one, look for ripe but still-firm fruit. Ripe peaches are incredibly tasty, but when diced and tossed with other ingredients, they tend to get mushy.

PER SERVING Calories: 37; Total fat: 0g; Saturated fat: 0g; Cholesterol: 0g; Sodium: 10g; Carbohydrates: 6g; Fiber: 1g; Phosphorus: 29mg; Potassium: 199mg; Protein: 1g

SOUR CREAM–DRESSED CUCUMBERS

Serves 4 / Prep time: 20 minutes (plus 1 hour chilling time)

LOW PROTEIN LOW FAT Cucumbers have a mild, fresh flavor that marries well with other ingredients like sour cream and dill. English cucumbers are the best choice, because they have a thin skin and very few seeds, unlike regular cucumbers, which can be bitter and seedy, especially if they are large. If you do use a regular cucumber, peel it first because the skin is often thick and covered with wax for transportation purposes.

2 tablespoons light sour cream

2 tablespoons plain yogurt

1 tablespoon apple cider vinegar

1½ teaspoons sugar

1 teaspoon chopped fresh dill

2 English cucumbers, cut into long ribbons with a vegetable peeler

1 scallion, white and green parts, chopped

1. In a large bowl, whisk together the sour cream, yogurt, vinegar, sugar, and dill until blended.

2. Add the cucumber and scallion, and toss to coat.

3. Refrigerate, covered, for at least 1 hour.

4. Stir and serve.

Cooking tip If you don't want to have to keep stirring this salad, to purge cucumber juices, you can drain the vegetables first. Place the cucumber ribbons in a sieve over the sink and rest a weight on them for at least 30 minutes to press out the excess juices.

PER SERVING Calories: 45; Total fat: 0g; Saturated fat: 0g; Cholesterol: 0mg; Sodium: 16mg; Carbohydrates: 9g; Fiber: 1g; Phosphorus: 50g; Potassium: 200mg; Protein: 1g

COBB SALAD

Serves 6 / Prep time: 15 minutes

Cobb salad is a famous creation from the 1930s, originating at the Brown Derby restaurant in Hollywood. This version is not exactly like the original, but features fresh, creamy avocado as a delectable topping. Avocado is a perfect accompaniment for the tomatoes because it can boost the body's absorption of lycopene, an antioxidant in tomatoes, by about 400 percent. Avocado can help lower cholesterol, reduce the risk of cardiovascular disease, and support liver health.

FOR THE DRESSING

¼ cup olive oil

3 tablespoons balsamic vinegar

1 teaspoon honey

1 teaspoon chopped fresh thyme

Freshly ground black pepper

FOR THE SALAD

6 cups mixed baby greens

1 cup halved cherry tomatoes

2 large hardboiled eggs, peeled and chopped

1 cup chopped cooked chicken breast

¼ ripe avocado, peeled, pitted, and diced

TO MAKE THE DRESSING

In a small bowl, whisk together the oil, balsamic vinegar, honey, and thyme and season with pepper. Set aside.

TO MAKE THE SALAD

1. In a large bowl, toss together the greens, cherry tomatoes, eggs, chicken, and avocado.

2. Arrange the salads on plates, and drizzle with the dressing. Serve.

Ingredient tip Premade cooked chicken is best when you make it yourself, rather than buying a rotisserie chicken or packaged cooked product, because those items contain a staggering amount of sodium. Cooking your own chicken breasts helps you control sodium levels. You can store cooked chicken in a sealed container in the refrigerator for up to 5 days.

PER SERVING Calories: 170; Total fat: 12g; Saturated fat: 2g; Cholesterol: 90mg; Sodium: 51mg; Carbohydrates: 5g; Fiber: 1g; Phosphorus: 103mg; Potassium: 200mg; Protein: 10g

CHICKEN CABBAGE SALAD

Serves 6 / Prep time: 20 minutes

The cabbage part of this dish is quite crunchy in itself, but the almonds provide extra texture and a rich nutty flavor. Almonds are the fruit of the almond tree, and are a stellar source of monounsaturated fats, which support a healthy cardiovascular system and reduce cholesterol. Almonds are also high in vitamin E, manganese, copper, and magnesium.

FOR THE DRESSING
½ cup Low-Sodium Mayonnaise (page 70)
2 tablespoons apple cider vinegar
1 teaspoon sugar
Freshly ground black pepper

FOR THE SALAD
4 cups finely shredded cabbage
¼ cup shredded carrot
2 scallions, white and green parts, julienned
1 cup chopped cooked chicken breast
2 tablespoons chopped fresh cilantro
2 tablespoons toasted slivered almonds

TO MAKE THE DRESSING

In a small bowl, whisk together the mayonnaise, vinegar, and sugar and season with pepper. Set aside.

TO MAKE THE SALAD

1. In a large bowl, toss together the cabbage, carrot, scallions, chicken, and cilantro.

2. Add the dressing to the salad, and toss to coat.

3. Top with the almonds, and serve.

Cooking tip This salad is a variation of coleslaw, a dish that gets better tasting as it sits. If you have the time, make the slaw portion of the salad and combine it with the dressing the day before you need it, and add the chicken, cilantro, and almonds just before serving.

PER SERVING Calories: 120; Total fat: 6g; Saturated fat: 1g; Cholesterol: 24mg; Sodium: 53mg; Carbohydrates: 8g; Fiber: 2g; Phosphorus: 86mg; Potassium: 200mg; Protein: 9g

GREEK COUSCOUS SALAD

Serves 5/ Prep time: 15 minutes

LOW PROTEIN LOW FAT This piquant summer salad can be served in any season, but it seems to belong on sunny patios, scooped onto paper plates with grilled burgers or spicy chicken breasts. Couscous is a simple grain to prepare, but if you prefer, white rice or bulgur can be substituted. If you swap out the couscous, just remember that this will also increase the potassium and phosphorus in each serving.

3 cups cooked couscous

1 English cucumber, diced

1 cup cherry tomatoes

1 scallion, white and green parts, chopped

½ cup quartered black olives

2 tablespoons chopped fresh parsley

2 tablespoons balsamic vinegar

1 tablespoon freshly squeezed lemon juice

¼ cup low-sodium feta cheese

1. In a large bowl, mix together the couscous, cucumber, tomatoes, scallion, olives, parsley, vinegar, and lemon juice.

2. Top the salad with the feta cheese, and serve.

Low-sodium tip Feta cheese is a staple ingredient in Greek cooking, but you can swap it with another cheese if you want to reduce the sodium. Low-sodium Parmesan cheese has just 18 mg sodium per ounce, and still imparts a nice strong flavor.

PER SERVING Calories: 116; Total fat: 3g; Saturated fat: 1g; Cholesterol: 7mg; Sodium: 164mg; Carbohydrates: 19g; Fiber: 2g; Phosphorus: 62mg; Potassium: 198mg; Protein: 4g

BULGUR VEGETABLE SALAD

Serves 5 / Prep time: 15 minutes

LOW PROTEIN LOW FAT Bulgur is a slightly chewy, nutty-tasting grain that does not get used enough in recipes, perhaps because people think it is difficult to cook. It is as simple as any other grain; just simmer it in water until tender, then drain. Bulgur is often found in Middle Eastern cuisines, and is high in fiber, iron, niacin, and zinc. This low-fat grain can help reduce inflammation and cut the risk of cancer and gallstones.

1 cup cooked bulgur

1 cup chopped broccoli

1 cup chopped cauliflower

1 red bell pepper, finely diced

1 scallion, white and green parts, chopped

2 tablespoons chopped fresh basil leaves

Juice and zest of 1 lemon

1 tablespoon olive oil

Freshly ground black pepper

1. In a large bowl, toss together the bulgur, broccoli, cauliflower, bell pepper, scallion, basil, lemon juice, lemon zest, and olive oil. Season with pepper.

2. Toss again and serve.

Ingredient tip Bulgur is usually carried in your grocery store where organic products are displayed. Look for cracked bulgur rather than whole, or you will have to double your cooking time.

PER SERVING Calories: 117; Total fat: 3g; Saturated fat: 0g; Cholesterol: 0mg; Sodium: 15mg; Carbohydrates: 21g; Fiber: 4g; Phosphorus: 59mg; Potassium: 199mg; Protein: 2g

CITRUS ORZO SALAD

Serves 4 / Prep time: 15 minutes

LOW PROTEIN You might be tempted to use the tart, slightly hot dressing for this salad in other recipes. The flavors here may feel a little Italian, which is logical because Italy has been the home of citrus fruit for more than 2,000 years. Countless citrus varieties grow in Italy, and both lemon and lime are prevalent in the cuisine of the region. Try adding a little orange zest as well, if you want a burst of sweetness.

FOR THE DRESSING
¼ cup olive oil
Juice of ½ lemon
Juice and zest of ½ lime
2 tablespoons grated Parmesan cheese
2 tablespoons chopped fresh oregano
¼ teaspoon red pepper flakes

FOR THE SALAD
3 cups cooked orzo pasta
1 yellow bell pepper, diced
1 red bell pepper, diced
½ small red onion, chopped
1 medium zucchini, diced

TO MAKE THE DRESSING

In a small bowl, whisk together the olive oil, lemon juice, lime juice, lime zest, Parmesan cheese, oregano, and red pepper flakes. Set aside.

TO MAKE THE SALAD

1. In a large bowl, toss together the orzo, yellow bell pepper, red bell pepper, onion, and zucchini.

2. Add the dressing, toss well to combine, and serve.

Ingredient tip Orzo is a small pasta that looks like rice or barley grains, and can create dishes that have a risotto-like texture. Orzo is made from the hard wheat berry, which ensures the pasta holds its shape and does not overcook easily.

PER SERVING Calories: 320; Total fat: 16g; Saturated fat: 2g; Cholesterol: 2mg; Sodium: 40mg; Carbohydrates: 33g; Fiber: 3g; Phosphorus: 33mg; Potassium: 107mg; Protein: 6g

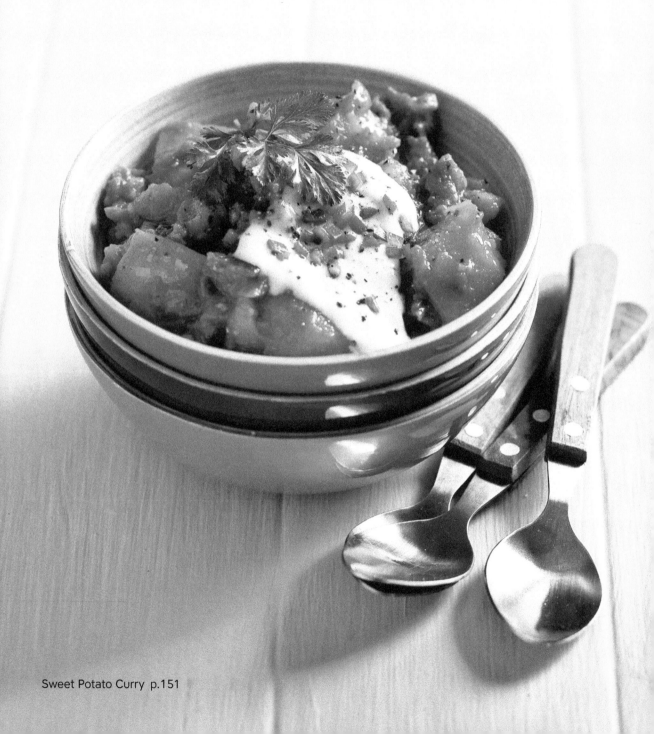

Sweet Potato Curry p.151

10

VEGETARIAN DISHES

BEAN VEGGIE TACOS

Serves 4 / Prep time: 30 minutes

LOW PROTEIN LOW FAT Tacos are messy, hard to hold, and lots of fun. If you want an even more festive meal, arrange the various fillings and toppings in bowls on the table, and let everyone put their tacos together themselves. Just watch your portion of beans if you need to limit your potassium—you can always use plenty of veggies instead, and maybe add a light scattering of cheese.

4 ounces sodium-free black beans, drained and rinsed

1 tablespoon freshly squeezed lime juice

½ jalapeño pepper, chopped

1 teaspoon chili powder

1 carrot, shredded

2 radishes, chopped

1 tablespoon chopped fresh cilantro

4 soft flour taco shells, warmed

2 cups shredded lettuce

1. In a blender, add the beans, lime juice, jalapeño pepper, and chili powder and pulse until coarsely chopped but still very chunky.

2. Transfer the bean mixture to a medium bowl, and stir in the carrot, radishes, and cilantro.

3. Spoon the bean-veggie mixture into the taco shells, and top each with lettuce.

Ingredient tip The taco shells in this dish are made with flour, not with corn. Corn taco shells have higher levels of potassium and phosphorus.

PER SERVING Calories: 108; Total fat: 3g; Saturated fat: 0g; Cholesterol: 0mg; Sodium: 23mg; Carbohydrates: 17g; Fiber: 4g; Phosphorus: 84mg; Potassium: 199mg; Protein: 4g

SWEET POTATO CURRY

Serves 6 / Prep time: 20 minutes / Cook time: 20 minutes

LOW PROTEIN Sweet potatoes are relatively high in potassium, but the level is within range when consumed in a relatively small portion, like this curry. Sweet potatoes are an excellent source of beta-carotene, fiber, vitamin A, and vitamin C. Although you are probably used to vibrant orange sweet potatoes, don't be surprised if you ever cut into one and find deep purple flesh. Purple sweet potatoes contain anthocyanins, which are powerful antioxidants.

2 teaspoons olive oil

1 medium sweet onion, chopped

1 tablespoon grated peeled fresh ginger

1 teaspoon minced fresh garlic

2 cups diced peeled sweet potatoes

1 cup diced carrots

1 cup water

½ cup heavy (whipping) cream

1 tablespoon curry powder

1 teaspoon ground cumin

2 tablespoons low-fat plain yogurt

2 tablespoons chopped fresh cilantro

1. In a large saucepan over medium-high heat, heat the olive oil.

2. Add the onion, ginger, and garlic and sauté until softened, about 3 minutes.

3. Add the sweet potatoes, carrots, water, cream, curry powder, and cumin and stir to mix well. Bring the mixture to a boil. Reduce the heat to low, and simmer until the vegetables are tender, about 15 minutes.

4. Serve immediately, topped with the yogurt and cilantro.

Substitution tip Almost any vegetable will work in a dish like curry, so let your creative impulses run wild. Stick to renal-friendly vegetables listed in this book (see Phosphorus, page 25, and Potassium, page 32) to ensure your mineral levels are within the correct range.

PER SERVING Calories: 132; Total fat: 9g; Saturated fat: 5g; Cholesterol: 27mg; Sodium: 40mg; Carbohydrates: 13g; Fiber: 2g; Phosphorus: 48mg; Potassium: 200mg; Protein: 1g

ZUCCHINI NOODLES WITH SPRING VEGETABLES

Serves 6 / Prep time: 20 minutes / Cook time: 10 minutes

LOW PROTEIN LOW FAT Fresh and supremely inviting might describe the way heaps of vegetable noodles, asparagus spears, and plump cherry tomatoes look on your plate. Since they are vegetables, these noodles do not taste a thing like pasta, but you can still wind them around a fork and suck them up like spaghetti. If you get a medium to large, firm zucchini, and you have a spiralizer (see Cooking tip), you can spin out strands that are several feet in length, so you might want to snip them shorter—or not! (If you don't have a spiralizer, you can use a vegetable peeler to create the veggie noodles.) Zucchini noodles can keep in the refrigerator for up to 3 days in a sealed container.

6 zucchini, cut into long noodles

1 cup halved snow peas

1 cup (3-inch pieces) asparagus

1 tablespoon olive oil

1 teaspoon minced fresh garlic

1 tablespoon freshly squeezed lemon juice

1 cup shredded fresh spinach

¾ cup halved cherry tomatoes

2 tablespoons chopped fresh basil leaves

1. Fill a medium saucepan with water, place over medium-high heat, and bring to a boil.

2. Reduce the heat to medium, and blanch the zucchini ribbons, snow peas, and asparagus by submerging them in the water for 1 minute. Drain and rinse immediately under cold water.

3. Pat the vegetables dry with paper towels, and transfer to a large bowl.

4. Place a medium skillet over medium heat, and add the olive oil. Add the garlic, and sauté until tender, about 3 minutes.

5. Add the lemon juice and spinach, and sauté until the spinach is wilted, about 3 minutes.

6. Add the zucchini mixture, the cherry tomatoes, and basil and toss until well combined.

7. Serve immediately.

Cooking tip A spiralizer is a good investment. This inexpensive culinary tool can create the most delightful long noodles from fruit and vegetables for an inventive presentation.

PER SERVING Calories: 52; Total fat: 2g; Saturated fat: 0g; Cholesterol: 0mg; Sodium: 7mg; Carbohydrates: 4g; Fiber: 1g; Phosphorus: 40mg; Potassium: 197mg; Protein: 2g

STIR-FRIED VEGETABLES

Serves 4/ Prep time: 15 minutes / Cook time: 15 minutes

LOW PROTEIN LOW FAT Broccoli is a base ingredient in many stir-fries because it cooks quickly and looks spectacular heaped with other vegetables with its tightly bunched florets. Broccoli is a cruciferous vegetable like cauliflower and cabbage, so it has the ability to lower cholesterol and detoxify the body. Broccoli can also help fight cancer. Be sure to not overcook this vegetable.

2 teaspoons olive oil

½ medium red onion, sliced

1 tablespoon grated peeled fresh ginger

2 teaspoons minced garlic

2 cups broccoli florets

2 cups cauliflower florets

1 red bell pepper, diced

1 cup sliced carrots

1. In a large skillet over medium-high heat, heat the olive oil.

2. Add the onion, ginger, and garlic and sauté until softened, about 3 minutes.

3. Add the broccoli, cauliflower, bell pepper, and carrots, and sauté until tender, about 10 minutes.

4. Serve hot.

Cooking tip This dish is great served over steaming white basmati rice to create a satisfying meal. Avoid brown rice if you are watching your phosphorus levels, because brown rice has twice as much phosphorus as white rice.

PER SERVING Calories: 50; Total fat: 1g; Saturated fat: 0g; Cholesterol: Ômg; Sodium: 26mg; Carbohydrates: 6g; Fiber: 2g; Phosphorus: 36mg; Potassium: 198mg; Protein: 1g

LIME ASPARAGUS SPAGHETTI

Serves 6 / Prep time: 5 minutes / Cook time: 20 minutes

LOW PROTEIN LOW FAT Asparagus has a fresh, almost grassy taste with a hint of sweetness, especially if you purchase the pencil-thin young asparagus. Part of the charm of this pretty salad is the long asparagus strips, which look like noodles. Asparagus is an excellent source of vitamin A, helping to support healthy eyes and reducing inflammation in the body.

1 pound asparagus spears, trimmed and cut into 2-inch pieces

2 teaspoons olive oil

2 teaspoons minced garlic

2 teaspoons all-purpose flour

1 cup Homemade Rice Milk (page 80, or use unsweetened store-bought) or almond milk

Juice and zest of ½ lemon

1 tablespoon chopped fresh thyme

Freshly ground black pepper

2 cups cooked spaghetti

¼ cup grated Parmesan cheese

1. Fill a large saucepan with water and bring to a boil over high heat. Add the asparagus and blanch until crisp-tender, about 2 minutes. Drain and set aside.

2. In a large skillet over medium-high heat, heat the olive oil. Add the garlic, and sauté until softened, about 2 minutes. Whisk in the flour to create a paste, about 1 minute. Whisk in the rice milk, lemon juice, lemon zest, and thyme.

3. Reduce the heat to medium and cook the sauce, whisking constantly, until thickened and creamy, about 3 minutes.

4. Season the sauce with pepper.

5. Stir in the spaghetti and the asparagus.

6. Serve the pasta topped with the Parmesan cheese.

Substitution tip Spaghetti looks lovely with the slender asparagus, but any pasta shape will work. Try farfalle, penne, or corkscrew cavatappi for this dish.

PER SERVING Calories: 127; Total fat: 3g; Saturated fat: 1g; Cholesterol: 4mg; Sodium: 67mg; Carbohydrates: 19g; Fiber: 2g; Phosphorus: 109mg; Potassium: 200mg; Protein: 6g

GARDEN CRUSTLESS QUICHE

Serves 6 / Prep time: 10 minutes / Cook time: 25 minutes

Kale is the darling of today's nutrition world because it is packed with fiber, vitamins, and minerals. One cup of kale has over 1,000 percent of the daily recommended amount of vitamin K and 100 percent of the recommended vitamin A. Kale is lower in potassium than other dark leafy greens and it's high in iron, which is often deficient in those with kidney problems. Try different varieties of kale, because the taste and appearance of the various species can vary.

6 eggs

2 egg whites

¼ cup Homemade Rice Milk (page 80; or use unsweetened store-bought)

¼ cup shredded Swiss cheese, divided

¼ teaspoon freshly ground black pepper

1 teaspoon unsalted butter, plus more for the pie plate

1 teaspoon minced garlic

1 scallion, white and green parts, chopped

1 yellow zucchini, chopped

½ cup shredded stemmed kale

1 cup quartered cherry tomatoes

1. In a medium bowl, beat the eggs, egg whites, rice milk, half the Swiss cheese, and the pepper until well blended, and set aside.

2. Preheat the oven to 350°F.

3. Grease a 9-inch pie plate with butter and set aside.

4. In a medium skillet over medium-high heat, melt 1 teaspoon of butter. Add the garlic and scallion, and sauté until softened, about 2 minutes.

5. Add the zucchini and kale, and sauté until wilted, about 3 minutes.

6. Transfer the vegetables from the skillet to the pie plate and add the tomatoes, spreading the vegetables evenly across the bottom.

7. Pour the egg mixture into the pie plate, and sprinkle with the remaining half of the Swiss cheese.

8. Bake until the quiche is puffed and lightly browned, 15 to 20 minutes.

9. Serve hot, warm, or cold.

Ingredient tip Yellow zucchini, sometimes called summer squash, is usually found lined up in a bin next to the more common green variety. You can interchange green with yellow in this dish.

PER SERVING Calories: 120; Total fat: 8g; Saturated fat: 4g; Cholesterol: 221mg; Sodium: 93mg; Carbohydrates: 3g; Fiber: 0g; Phosphorus: 120mg; Potassium: 189mg; Protein: 9g

LENTIL VEGGIE BURGERS

Serves 4 / Prep time: 15 minutes (plus 1 hour chilling time) / Cook time: 10 minutes

LOW FAT This underestimated familiar green is actually an incredible diuretic and very effective heavy metal detoxifier. Consuming parsley as part of your regular diet can reduce the risk of kidney stones and help treat existing urinary tract infections. Either flat leaf or curly leaf parsley will do the trick, because they taste almost the same and have an identical nutrition profile.

2½ cups cooked white rice

½ cup cooked red lentils, drained and rinsed

2 eggs, lightly beaten

2 tablespoons chopped fresh parsley

2 teaspoons chopped fresh basil leaves

Juice and zest of 1 lime

1 teaspoon minced garlic

1 tablespoon olive oil

1. In a food processor (or blender), pulse the rice, lentils, eggs, parsley, basil, lime juice, lime zest, and garlic until the mixture holds together.

2. Transfer the rice mixture to a medium bowl, and set in the refrigerator until it firms up, about 1 hour.

3. Form the rice mixture into 4 patties.

4. In a large skillet over medium-high heat, heat the olive oil.

5. Add the veggie patties and cook until golden, about 5 minutes. Flip the patties over. Cook the other side for 5 minutes.

6. Transfer the burgers to a paper towel–lined plate.

7. Serve the veggie burgers hot with your favorite toppings.

Substitution tip Veggie burgers can be made with many types of legumes as the base, like the red lentils used in this version. Chickpeas, navy beans, pinto beans, and split peas can all be substituted for the lentils in the same amount.

PER SERVING Calories: 247; Total fat: 7g; Saturated fat: 2g; Cholesterol: 106mg; Sodium: 36mg; Carbohydrates: 31g; Fiber: 3g; Phosphorus: 120mg; Potassium: 183mg; Protein: 8g

BAKED CAULIFLOWER RICE CAKES

Serves 6 / Prep time: 10 minutes / Cook time: 20 minutes

A passerby might mistake these golden nuggets for unusual muffins because they are the same shape, but the savory cheesy taste of the rice cakes is unmistakable. From this recipe, one portion of the cooked rice, tender cauliflower, and creamy yogurt combination will fill you up easily, and is satisfying paired with a green salad.

Olive oil for the pan
2 cups chopped blanched cauliflower
   (see Cooking tip)
2 cups cooked white basmati rice
¼ cup plain yogurt

2 eggs, lightly beaten
½ cup grated Cheddar cheese
¼ teaspoon ground nutmeg
Freshly ground black pepper

1. Preheat the oven to 350°F.

2. Lightly coat 6 cups of a standard muffin tin with olive oil.

3. In a large bowl, mix together the cauliflower, rice, yogurt, eggs, cheese, and nutmeg.

4. Season the mixture with pepper.

5. Evenly divide the cauliflower mixture among the 6 prepared muffin cups.

6. Bake until golden and slightly puffy, about 20 minutes.

7. Let them stand for 5 minutes, then run a knife around the edges to loosen.

8. Serve hot, warm, or cold.

Cooking tip To blanch the chopped cauliflower, plunge into boiling water for 3 minutes, then drain and rinse with cold water.

PER SERVING Calories: 141; Total fat: 5g; Saturated fat: 3g; Cholesterol: 82mg; Sodium: 98mg; Carbohydrates: 18g; Fiber: 1g; Phosphorus: 119mg; Potassium: 178mg; Protein: 7g

VEGETABLE RICE CASSEROLE

Serves 4 / Prep time: 10 minutes / Cook time: 50 minutes

LOW FAT Vegetarian dishes do not have to be complicated to be delicious. People often underestimate the unfussy recipes—there's no need to sprout your own alfalfa or press your own tofu. This recipe makes that point, with rice, vegetables, and a little sprinkle of cheese, which combine to create a perfect midweek meal or quick lunch when you need a little extra energy. Have some fun testing out all types of vegetables for different variations.

1 teaspoon olive oil

½ small sweet onion, chopped

½ teaspoon minced garlic

½ cup chopped red bell pepper

1 cup chopped fresh green beans

¼ cup grated carrot

1 cup white basmati rice

2 cups water

¼ cup grated Parmesan cheese

Freshly ground black pepper

1. Preheat the oven to 350°F.

2. In a medium skillet over medium-high heat, heat the olive oil.

3. Add the onion and garlic, and sauté until softened, about 3 minutes.

4. Add the bell pepper, green beans, and carrot, and sauté for 2 minutes.

5. Transfer the vegetables to a 9-by-9-inch baking dish, and stir in the rice and water.

6. Cover the dish and bake until the liquid is absorbed, 35 to 40 minutes.

7. Sprinkle the cheese on top and bake an additional 5 minutes to melt.

8. Season the casserole with pepper, and serve.

Substitution tip Not surprisingly, the cheesy topping on this casserole elevates it to a truly sublime experience. You can also try feta, Cheddar cheese, and goat cheese for different tastes and textures.

PER SERVING Calories: 224; Total fat: 3g; Saturated fat: 1g; Cholesterol: 6mg; Sodium: 105mg; Carbohydrates: 41g; Fiber: 2g; Phosphorus: 118mg; Potassium: 176mg; Protein: 6g

EGG FRIED RICE

Serves 6 / Prep time: 10 minutes / Cook time: 20 minutes

This robust version of the familiar restaurant fare is more Indonesian and is close to a traditional dish called nasi goreng (fried rice), which uses limited oil and includes fresh vegetables and egg. The egg in nasi goreng is often fried sunny-side up and placed over the finished rice, but as is directed here, scrambled works well too.

1 tablespoon olive oil

1 tablespoon grated peeled fresh ginger

1 teaspoon minced garlic

1 cup chopped carrots

1 scallion, white and green parts, chopped

2 tablespoons chopped fresh cilantro

4 cups cooked rice

1 tablespoon low-sodium soy sauce

4 eggs, beaten

1. In a large skillet over medium-high heat, heat the olive oil.

2. Add the ginger and garlic, and sauté until softened, about 3 minutes.

3. Add the carrots, scallion, and cilantro, and sauté until tender, about 5 minutes.

4. Stir in the rice and soy sauce, and sauté until the rice is heated through, about 5 minutes.

5. Move the rice over to one side of the skillet, and pour the eggs into the empty space.

6. Scramble the eggs, then mix them into the rice.

7. Serve hot.

Low-sodium tip Soy sauces, even low-sodium versions, are very salty. If you have the time, making your own substitution sauce is simple and effective, even if it does not taste quite the same. There are many versions of this diet-friendly sauce online, with ingredients like vinegar, molasses, garlic, and herbs.

PER SERVING Calories: 204; Total fat: 6g; Saturated fat: 1g; Cholesterol: 141mg; Sodium: 223mg; Carbohydrates: 29g; Fiber: 1g; Phosphorus: 120mg; Potassium: 147mg; Protein: 8g

MUSHROOM RICE NOODLES

Serves 4 / Prep time: 15 minutes / Cook time: 15 minutes

LOW PROTEIN LOW FAT Rice noodles come in an assortment of types and are the foundation for many classic Asian dishes such as pad Thai and pho. You will be confronted by packages of Asian noodles when trying to pick out the ones for this recipe, with options such as udon, soba, and lo mein. Look for plain rice noodles that are transparent and about ¼ inch wide. If you get the other variations, then the nutrition data will change, because they have added ingredients like buckwheat.

4 cups rice noodles

2 teaspoons toasted sesame oil

2 cups sliced wild mushrooms

2 teaspoons minced garlic

1 red bell pepper, sliced

1 yellow bell pepper, sliced

1 carrot, julienned

2 scallions, white and green parts, sliced

1 tablespoon low-sodium soy sauce

1. Prepare the rice noodles according to the package instructions and set them aside.

2. In a large skillet over medium-high heat, heat the sesame oil.

3. Add the mushrooms and garlic, and sauté until lightly caramelized, about 7 minutes.

4. Sauté the red bell pepper, yellow bell pepper, carrot, and scallions until tender, about 5 minutes.

5. Stir in the soy sauce and rice noodles, and toss to coat.

6. Serve.

Low-sodium tip Liquid aminos or coconut aminos—a sauce usually shelved near the soy sauce in supermarkets—is a reasonable substitute for soy sauce, at about 360 mg per tablespoon. Regular soy sauce has approximately 920 mg of sodium per tablespoon and low-sodium soy sauce has approximately 575 mg per tablespoon.

PER SERVING Calories: 163; Total fat: 2g; Saturated fat: 0g; Cholesterol: 0mg; Sodium: 199mg; Carbohydrates: 33g; Fiber: 2g; Phosphorus: 69mg; Potassium: 200mg; Protein: 2g

MIXED VEGETABLE BARLEY

Serves 6 / Prep time: 15 minutes / Cook time: 35 minutes

LOW PROTEIN LOW FAT Barley is a cereal grain often found in soups because it adds substance, thickens the broth a little, and has a pleasing chewy texture. Very high in manganese, molybdenum, selenium, and fiber, barley is a good choice for regulating the digestive system and lowering cholesterol, as well as reducing the risk of cardiovascular disease. Either pearl barley or pot barley will yield the best results in this recipe.

1 tablespoon olive oil

1 medium sweet onion, chopped

2 teaspoons minced garlic

2 cups fresh cauliflower florets

1 red bell pepper, diced

1 carrot, sliced

½ cup barley

½ cup white rice

2 cups water

1 tablespoon minced fresh parsley

1. In a large skillet over medium-high heat, heat the olive oil.

2. Add the onion and garlic, and sauté until softened, about 3 minutes.

3. Stir in the cauliflower, bell pepper, and carrot, and sauté for 5 minutes.

4. Stir in the barley, rice, and water and bring to a boil.

5. Reduce the heat to low, cover, and simmer until the liquid is absorbed and the barley and rice are tender, about 25 minutes.

6. Serve topped with the parsley.

Cooking tip You can bake this dish in the oven rather than cooking it on the stove, and set it up completely the night before. Just transfer the sautéed vegetables to an 8-by-8-inch casserole dish and stir in the barley, rice, and water. Store in the refrigerator until ready to bake.

PER SERVING Calories: 156; Total fat: 3g; Saturated fat: 0g; Cholesterol: 0mg; Sodium: 16mg; Carbohydrates: 30g; Fiber: 4g; Phosphorus: 83mg; Potassium: 220mg; Protein: 4g

SPICY SESAME TOFU

Serves 6 / Prep time: 15 minutes / Cook time: 10 minutes

LOW PROTEIN LOW FAT Dedicated vegetarians sometimes walk right past the tofu display in the supermarket because they have no idea how to prepare these blocks of pressed soy. Tofu is made in a similar technique as cheese, so you can purchase tofu from soft all the way to extra firm, depending on how much liquid has been pressed out. Tofu is an amazing ingredient because it soaks up whatever flavors you add to it, and it can cook up crispy and firm. The sesame, ginger, soy sauce, and hot red pepper flakes in this dish combine to create a truly sublime blend for infusing the tofu.

1 tablespoon toasted sesame oil

1 tablespoon grated peeled fresh ginger

2 teaspoons minced garlic

2 red bell peppers, thinly sliced

1 (14-ounce) package extra-firm tofu, drained and cut into 1-inch cubes

2 cups quartered bok choy

2 scallions, white and green parts, cut thinly on a bias

3 tablespoons low-sodium soy sauce

2 tablespoons freshly squeezed lime juice

Pinch red pepper flakes

2 tablespoons chopped fresh cilantro

2 tablespoons toasted sesame seeds

1. In a large skillet over medium-high heat, heat the sesame oil.

2. Add the ginger and garlic, and sauté until softened, about 3 minutes.

3. Stir in the bell peppers and tofu, and gently sauté for about 3 minutes.

4. Add the bok choy and scallions, and sauté until the bok choy is wilted, about 3 minutes.

5. Add the soy sauce, lime juice, and red pepper flakes and toss to coat.

6. Serve topped with the cilantro and sesame seeds.

Low-sodium tip Almost all the sodium in this dish comes from the soy sauce, so reducing it or omitting it will significantly drop the amount of sodium per serving. The taste of the recipe will not be as strong, but using just 1 tablespoon of soy sauce in this recipe will create a serving with about 160 mg sodium.

PER SERVING Calories: 80; Total fat: 3g; Saturated fat: 0g; Cholesterol: 0mg; Sodium: 503mg; Carbohydrates: 4g; Fiber: 1g; Phosphorus: 88mg; Potassium: 165mg; Protein: 6g

TOFU HOISIN SAUTÉ

Serves 4 / Prep time: 15 minutes / Cook time: 20 minutes

If you are a fan of spicy, hot food, this will please your palate. A whole jalapeño pepper is used to create a complex heat that is not overwhelmingly mouth-scorching. If you want a relatively mild pepper, look for one that is green rather than red, and avoid peppers with white striations running lengthwise down the sides. These striations indicate that the pepper is older, which equates to infinitely hotter.

2 tablespoons hoisin sauce

2 tablespoons rice vinegar

1 teaspoon cornstarch

2 tablespoons olive oil

1 (15-ounce) package extra-firm tofu, cut into 1-inch cubes

2 cups unpeeled cubed eggplant

2 scallions, white and green parts, sliced

2 teaspoons minced garlic

1 jalapeño pepper, minced

2 tablespoons chopped fresh cilantro

1. In a small bowl, whisk together the hoisin sauce, rice vinegar, and cornstarch and set aside.

2. In a large skillet over medium-high heat, heat the olive oil. Add the tofu, and sauté gently until golden brown, about 10 minutes, and transfer to a plate.

3. Reduce the heat to medium. Add the eggplant, scallions, garlic, and jalapeño pepper, and sauté until tender and fragrant, about 6 minutes.

4. Stir in the reserved sauce, and toss until the sauce thickens, about 2 minutes.

5. Stir in the tofu and cilantro, and serve hot.

Low-sodium tip Hoisin sauce is made with soy sauce, so it does contain a hefty amount of sodium per serving. This recipe would still be tasty, while slightly less intensely flavored, if you use 1 tablespoon of hoisin sauce instead of 2 tablespoons.

PER SERVING Calories: 105; Total fat: 4g; Saturated fat: 1g; Cholesterol: 0mg; Sodium: 234mg; Carbohydrates: 9g; Fiber: 2g; Phosphorus: 105mg; Potassium: 192mg; Protein: 8g

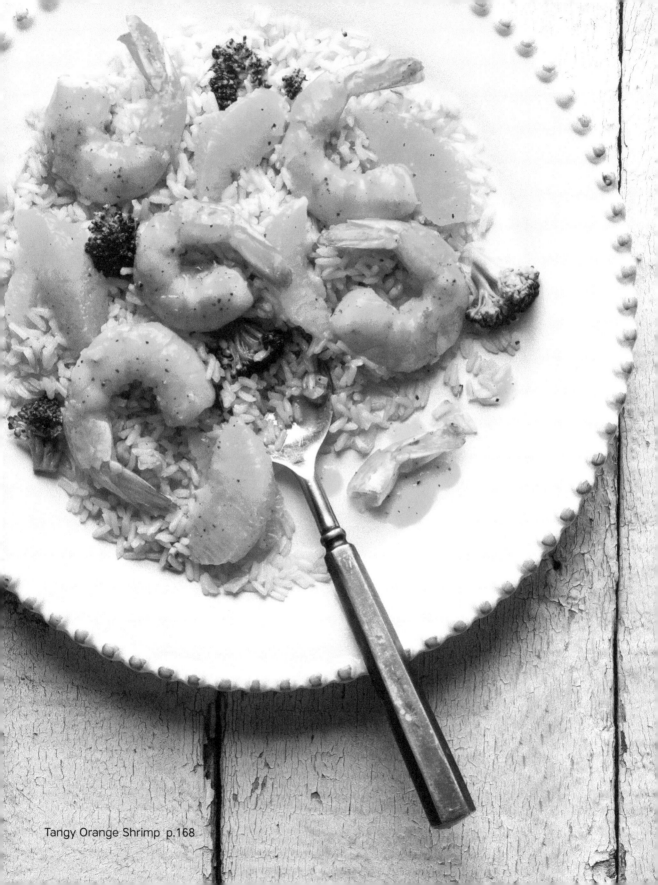

Tangy Orange Shrimp p.168

11

SEAFOOD DISHES

TANGY ORANGE SHRIMP

Serves 4 / Prep time: 15 minutes / Cook time: 15 minutes

LOW FAT Delicate-looking pink shrimp look so inviting in this delectable orange sauce accompanied by bright broccoli spears. Try serving this dish over couscous or white basmati rice, because the sauce will soak into the grain beautifully.

½ cup freshly squeezed orange juice

½ teaspoon cornstarch

¼ teaspoon freshly grated orange zest

1 teaspoon olive oil

12 ounces (26/30 count) shrimp, peeled and deveined, tails left on

1 cup broccoli florets

1 teaspoon unsalted butter

½ cup orange segments (see Cooking tip)

Freshly ground black pepper

1. In a small bowl, whisk together the orange juice, cornstarch, and orange zest and set aside.

2. In a large skillet over medium-high heat, heat the olive oil.

3. Add the shrimp and sauté until just cooked through and opaque, about 5 minutes. Transfer the cooked shrimp to a plate. Add the broccoli and sauté until tender, about 4 minutes. Transfer to the plate with the shrimp.

4. Pour the orange juice mixture into the skillet, and whisk until the sauce has thickened and is glossy, about 3 minutes.

5. Whisk in the butter, and add the orange segments, shrimp, and broccoli to the skillet.

6. Toss to combine, and season with pepper. Serve immediately.

Cooking tip Segmenting oranges is different from just separating the membranes—you don't want the membranes at all—but it's easier than you might think. Cut the peel and pith off an orange, and use a paring knife to cut the segments out, following the membranes of the orange. Or you can use canned mandarin orange segments, which you can find in the supermarket.

PER SERVING Calories: 140; Total fat: 3g; Saturated fat: 1g; Cholesterol: 130g; Sodium: 132mg; Carbohydrates: 8g; Fiber: 1g; Phosphorus: 196mg; Potassium: 329mg; Protein: 18g

SHRIMP AND GREENS

Serves 4 / Prep time: 10 minutes / Cook time: 15 minutes

A fine dining establishment would be proud to serve this professional-looking dish, and the kitchen would be delighted to prepare it because it is so simple. Cherry tomatoes provide a burst of color to the dish and a heap of nutritional benefits. Tomatoes contain fiber, vitamins A, C, and K, and lycopene, a phytonutrient linked to cancer prevention and reduced risk of cardiovascular disease.

1 tablespoon olive oil

12 ounces (26/30 count) shrimp, peeled, deveined, tails removed

2 teaspoons minced garlic

2 cups fresh spinach

½ cup halved cherry tomatoes

½ teaspoon ground nutmeg

Freshly ground black pepper

1. In a large skillet over medium-high heat, heat the olive oil.

2. Add the shrimp and sauté until opaque and pink, about 6 minutes.

3. With a slotted spoon, remove the shrimp to a plate.

4. In the skillet, sauté the garlic until softened, about 3 minutes.

5. Stir in the spinach and tomatoes, and sauté until the spinach has wilted and the tomatoes are cooked, about 5 minutes.

6. Stir in the shrimp, sprinkle in the nutmeg, and toss to combine.

7. Season with pepper, and serve.

Cooking tip This recipe could easily be a topping for a rice noodle dish rather than an entrée by itself. Toss the finished dish with 2 cups of cooked rice noodles, and serve for a more substantial meal.

PER SERVING Calories: 127; Total fat: 8g; Saturated fat: 1g; Cholesterol: 85mg; Sodium: 96mg; Carbohydrates: 2g; Fiber: 1g; Phosphorus: 178mg; Potassium: 287mg; Protein: 18g

SEARED HERBED SCALLOPS

Serves 4 / Prep time: 15 minutes / Cook time: 5 minutes

Scallops are sweet and mouthwateringly tender when cooked right. They are not difficult to cook, but if you happen to overcook them then you will be left looking at pretty mollusks with the consistency of rubber. So, resist any urge to turn the heat up too high, and be sure to turn them after a couple of minutes so the center is still translucent and the sides are golden brown.

1 tablespoon olive oil
12 ounces sea scallops, rinsed and
   patted dry
Freshly ground black pepper

2 tablespoons freshly squeezed
   lemon juice
1 teaspoon chopped fresh parsley
1 teaspoon chopped fresh thyme
1 teaspoon chopped fresh chives

1. In a large skillet over medium-high heat, heat the olive oil.

2. Lightly season the scallops with pepper. Add them to the skillet.

3. Sear the scallops, turning once, until just cooked through and browned, about 4 minutes total.

4. Stir in the lemon juice, parsley, thyme, and chives.

5. Turn the scallops to coat in the herb sauce.

6. Serve hot.

Ingredient tip Sea scallops are best fresh, right out of the local fishmonger's counter, but you can find fine-quality frozen scallops, as well. Look for scallops that were flash-frozen right on the boat for the best quality.

PER SERVING Calories: 131; Total fat: 5g; Saturated fat: 1g; Cholesterol: 35mg; Sodium: 136mg; Carbohydrates: 2g; Fiber: 0g; Phosphorus: 176mg; Potassium: 268mg; Protein: 14g

ALMOND-CRUSTED SOLE

Serves 4 / Prep time: 15 minutes / Cook time: 15 minutes

LOW FAT You probably won't get the chance to see the strange appearance of the whole sole fish when you buy prepared fillets, but sole is a type of flatfish, which means its eyes are not where you would expect them to be, on either side—rather, both eyes are on the upper side. Sole should have a fresh, nonfishy odor, so make sure you ask to smell the fillets before purchasing them from a fish counter. The texture is very delicate and should not be mushy when pressed lightly with your fingertip. When in doubt, pick up a reputable frozen product that has been flash frozen.

4 (3-ounce) sole fillets, patted dry

Freshly ground black pepper

3 tablespoons almond flour

1 tablespoon chopped fresh parsley

1 teaspoon chopped fresh thyme

1 teaspoon olive oil

1. Preheat the oven to 350°F.

2. Line a baking sheet with parchment paper.

3. Lightly season the sole fillets with pepper.

4. In a shallow bowl, mix together the almond flour, parsley, and thyme until blended.

5. Lightly brush the fish with the olive oil, and dredge in the almond flour mixture.

6. Place the sole fillets on the prepared baking sheet, and bake until the fish is opaque, about 15 minutes.

7. Serve immediately.

Ingredient tip Black pepper is something most people are used to seeing in shakers on the table and the taste is very familiar. However, pepper can go stale and lose potency, so the best way to enjoy it is to fill your pepper grinder with black peppercorns and freshly grind your own pepper as needed.

PER SERVING Calories: 113; Total fat: 3g; Saturated fat: 1g; Cholesterol: 41mg; Sodium: 70mg; Carbohydrates: 1g; Fiber: 0g; Phosphorus: 168mg; Potassium: 327mg; Protein: 17g

BREADED BAKED SOLE

Serves 4 / Prep time: 10 minutes / Cook time: 10 minutes

LOW PROTEIN LOW FAT Breading fish or any other item can be a tedious and messy job. You might end up with breaded fingers as well, from all the dredging and dipping. This recipe offers a quick breading method that just presses the buttered bread crumbs on top of the fish in an even layer rather than encasing it. This means less scattered flour and crumbs on your counter, and a quicker prep time—you can complete this job in less than 10 minutes.

¼ cup bread crumbs

1 tablespoon unsalted butter,
   at room temperature

2 teaspoons chopped fresh parsley

2 teaspoons chopped fresh thyme

2 teaspoons freshly grated lemon zest

4 (2-ounce) sole fillets, skinless, patted dry

Freshly ground black pepper

1. Preheat the oven to 400°F.

2. In a small bowl, stir together the bread crumbs, butter, parsley, thyme, and lemon zest.

3. Lightly season the fish fillets with pepper, and place them on a baking sheet.

4. Divide the bread crumb mixture evenly among the fillets, pressing it down lightly to adhere.

5. Bake until the fish is just cooked through and the bread crumbs are golden, about 10 minutes.

Cooking tip This convenient recipe takes very little time to cook, and can be assembled and placed in the refrigerator or freezer until ready to bake. The fish can be baked right from frozen—just add 15 minutes to the cook time.

PER SERVING Calories: 103; Total fat: 3g; Saturated fat: 2g; Cholesterol: 35mg; Sodium: 96mg; Carbohydrates: 5g; Fiber: 0g; Phosphorus: 116mg; Potassium: 200mg; Protein: 8g

ROASTED TILAPIA WITH GARLIC BUTTER

Serves 4 / Prep time: 10 minutes / Cook time: 10 minutes

For people who want to eat healthy, garlic butter is one of those decadent sauces destined to be a special treat rather than an everyday indulgence. Baking the fish right in the sauce makes the flesh incredibly tender and rich, so definitely serve this with a simple vegetable side dish or salad. Any white fish will work here, including sole, haddock, and halibut.

¼ cup melted unsalted butter

1 shallot, minced

1 teaspoon minced garlic

Juice and zest of ½ lemon

2 tablespoons chopped fresh parsley

1 tablespoon all-purpose flour

1 tablespoon olive oil

4 (3-ounce) tilapia fillets, patted dry

Freshly ground black pepper

1. Preheat the oven to 400°F.

2. In a small bowl, stir together the butter, shallot, garlic, lemon juice, lemon zest, parsley, and flour and set aside.

3. In a large ovenproof skillet over medium-high heat, heat the oil. Season the fillets with pepper and set them in the skillet. Brown the fish, turning once, about 4 minutes total.

4. Pour the butter mixture over the fish, and place the skillet, uncovered, in the oven. Roast the fish until just cooked through and opaque in the center, about 4 minutes.

5. Serve immediately with a spoonful of sauce from the skillet.

Substitution tip Onion or scallion can be substituted for the shallot in the sauce. Shallot has a lighter, sweeter flavor.

PER SERVING Calories: 219; Total fat: 16g; Saturated fat: 8g; Cholesterol: 72mg; Sodium: 45mg; Carbohydrates: 2g; Fiber: 0g; Phosphorus: 149mg; Potassium: 252mg; Protein: 17g

PESTO-CRUSTED TILAPIA

Serves 4 / Prep time: 10 minutes / Cook time: 15 minutes

LOW FAT Anything "crusted" seems to evoke a mouthwatering response. And pesto is a condiment that combines well with almost any meal ingredient. Pesto can top any type of protein from steak to fish. It can be spooned into soups, and tossed with pasta or vegetables. If you enjoy pesto, it might be cost-efficient to make your own from a favorite recipe rather than buy prepared products. You can also control the sodium and other nutritional elements with homemade pesto.

Olive oil, for the baking dish
½ cup bread crumbs
1 tablespoon grated Parmesan cheese

1 tablespoon Basil Pesto (page 67)
4 (3-ounce) tilapia fillets, patted dry

1. Preheat the oven to 400°F.
2. Lightly coat a 9-by-9-inch baking dish with olive oil, and set it aside.
3. In a small bowl, add the bread crumbs, Parmesan cheese, and pesto and stir until blended.
4. Place the fish in the baking dish, and spoon the pesto mixture over the fish so each piece is evenly coated.
5. Bake until just cooked through, about 15 minutes.
6. Serve hot.

Cooking tip If you have a barbecue, this recipe is perfect for cooking outdoors on a balmy summer evening. Turn one side of your barbecue on high, and leave the other side off. Place the fish in a foil package instead of a baking dish, on the cool side of the barbecue, for about 25 minutes.

PER SERVING Calories: 159; Total fat: 5g; Saturated fat: 1g; Cholesterol: 43mg; Sodium: 162mg; Carbohydrates: 10g; Fiber: 1g; Phosphorus: 164mg; Potassium: 272mg; Protein: 19g

LIME BAKED HADDOCK

Serves 4 / Prep time: 10 minutes / Cook time: 10 minutes

Limes look like little green lemons, and they come from the same family as their bigger yellow cousins, but limes have a unique taste that enhances the fish in this dish. Baking the fish directly on sliced limes is a healthy option because the pith—the white section between the flesh and rind—contains high amounts of limonene, a powerful phytonutrient. Limes can help reduce the risk of cancer and are an efficient detoxifier, important for kidney health.

4 (3-ounce) haddock fillets, patted dry

Freshly ground black pepper

Olive oil cooking spray

3 limes, thinly sliced

1 tablespoon olive oil

3 tablespoons crushed almonds

2 teaspoons chopped fresh dill

1. Preheat the oven to 400°F.

2. Lightly season the fish with pepper.

3. Lightly coat a 9-by-9-inch baking dish with cooking spray.

4. Lay the lime slices in the bottom of the baking dish, and arrange the fish fillets on top.

5. Brush the fish with the olive oil, and sprinkle them with the almonds.

6. Bake the fish until just cooked through and the almonds are golden, about 10 minutes.

7. Serve with the chopped dill.

Substitution tip Adding nuts to fish helps preserve moisture and infuses the fish with a lush, rich flavor. You can try cashews, walnuts, pistachios, hazelnuts, and any other favorite nuts until you hit upon the one that best suits your palate.

PER SERVING Calories: 124; Total fat: 6g; Saturated fat: 0g; Cholesterol: 55mg; Sodium: 59mg; Carbohydrates: 1g; Fiber: 0g; Phosphorus: 176mg; Potassium: 283mg; Protein: 17g

FISH TACOS WITH VEGETABLE SLAW

Serves 4 / Prep time: 20 minutes (plus 1 hour chilling time)

LOW PROTEIN LOW FAT Fish tacos are very popular on the West Coast because of the area's access to incredible seafood and a lifestyle that supports hand-held foods eaten on the run. You would be amazed at the variety of tacos available right on the beach in many areas of California. Any firm-flesh fish such as salmon, haddock, or sea bass would be luscious with the fresh salsa and mild tortilla.

FOR THE SLAW

2 cups finely shredded red cabbage

1 carrot, shredded

3 radishes, grated

2 tablespoons apple cider vinegar

Juice of 1 lime

1 teaspoon honey

1 teaspoon chopped fresh cilantro

FOR THE TACOS

4 (6-inch) flour tortillas

8 ounces halibut fillet, cooked

TO MAKE THE SLAW

1. In a medium bowl, toss together the cabbage, carrot, radishes, vinegar, lime juice, honey, and cilantro until well mixed.

2. Place the bowl in the refrigerator for 1 hour to let the flavors mellow.

TO MAKE THE TACOS

1. Place the tortillas on a clean work surface. Divide the fish evenly among them, then top with the slaw.

2. Fold the tortillas over the fish and serve.

Substitution tip Most commercially prepared fish tacos use soft tortillas, but you can use a crisp corn taco shell instead. With this change, you can cut the phosphorus and potassium by about 10 mg each per serving.

PER SERVING Calories: 131; Total fat: 3g; Saturated fat: 1g; Cholesterol: 32mg; Sodium: 57mg; Carbohydrates: 13g; Fiber: 2g; Phosphorus: 144mg; Potassium: 307mg; Protein: 12g

SALMON IN FOIL PACKETS

Serves 4 / Prep time: 10 minutes / Cook time: 20 minutes

LOW FAT Cooking individual portions in snug foil packets produces very flavorful, moist fish, because the juices get trapped in the packet and the fish basically steams. Be careful when you open the packet to check the fish or serve—the escaping steam can burn your fingers. Use kitchen tongs to pry open the top, and let the packet sit a minute before handling this tasty treat.

2 cups bean sprouts

1 red bell pepper, sliced

8 asparagus spears, cut into 2-inch pieces

1 scallion, white and green parts, chopped

4 (2-ounce) salmon fillets, skinless

Juice of 1 lemon

2 teaspoons grated peeled fresh ginger

1. Preheat the oven to 400°F.

2. Cut four pieces of foil, each about 12 inches square.

3. Divide the bean sprouts, bell pepper, asparagus, and scallion evenly and place on the foil pieces.

4. Place a salmon fillet on top of each pile of vegetables.

5. In a small bowl, stir together the lemon juice and ginger until well mixed.

6. Pour the ginger mixture evenly among the servings.

7. Fold the foil up into sealed packets and place them on a baking sheet.

8. Bake until the fish flakes when pressed with a fork, about 20 minutes.

9. Serve hot.

Cooking tip If you have a knack for folding paper, try using parchment paper instead of foil for this recipe. Parchment paper is the more traditional medium for cooking *en papillote*, and you can place the cooked packet right on the plate, and cut open to serve.

PER SERVING Calories: 119; Total fat: 6g; Saturated fat: 2g; Cholesterol: 28mg; Sodium: 29mg; Carbohydrates: 4g; Fiber: 1g; Phosphorus: 183mg; Potassium: 341mg; Protein: 13g

LEMON POACHED SALMON

Serves 4 / Prep time: 5 minutes / Cook time: 15 minutes

You might want to double or even triple this recipe and save the leftovers for another meal. This poached fish can be repurposed to make a tasty salmon salad, placed in chunks over a green salad, or even added to scrambled eggs or a baked egg dish. Poached salmon will keep in a sealed container in the refrigerator for up to 3 days.

1 cup water

Juice and zest of 1 lemon

2 tablespoons chopped fresh thyme

1 tablespoon chopped fresh dill

6 peppercorns

4 (3-ounce) skinless salmon fillets

1. In a large skillet over medium-high heat, add the water, lemon juice, lemon zest, thyme, dill, and peppercorns. Bring the liquid to a boil, then reduce the heat to low and simmer. Add the salmon fillets to the skillet and cover.

2. Poach the salmon until opaque and cooked through, about 15 minutes.

3. Transfer the salmon to a plate, and discard the poaching liquid.

4. Serve the fish hot or cold.

Ingredient tip You are probably used to the hard black peppercorns poured into grinders in fine restaurants, or maybe you have one of your own at home. Peppercorns can also be found in other colors, such as white and pretty pink, so try different peppercorns for a unique poaching liquid for the salmon in this dish.

PER SERVING Calories: 150; Total fat: 9g; Saturated fat: 3g; Cholesterol: 42mg; Sodium: 39mg; Carbohydrates: 0g; Fiber: 0g; Phosphorus: 243mg; Potassium: 331mg; Protein: 17g

SALMON WITH GREEN VEGETABLES

Serves 4 / Prep time: 10 minutes / Cook time: 20 minutes

LOW FAT Fish is one of the quickest meals to prepare and cook, which makes it attractive on busy days or when you have evening plans. Regardless, this dish tastes like it took some time to prepare, so enjoy its fresh decadence.

1 tablespoon olive oil, plus more for the baking dish

4 (2-ounce) boneless skinless salmon fillets

Freshly ground black pepper

1 cup (2-inch pieces) asparagus spears

1 cup quartered bok choy

2 tablespoons chopped fresh dill

Juice and zest of 1 lemon

1. Preheat the oven to 375°F.

2. Lightly coat a 9-by-9-inch baking dish with olive oil.

3. Lightly season the fish with pepper.

4. In the prepared baking dish, arrange the asparagus, bok choy, and dill, and top the vegetables with the fish fillets.

5. Sprinkle the lemon juice and lemon zest on the fish, and drizzle 1 tablespoon of olive oil over the salmon and vegetables.

6. Cover the dish with foil, and bake until the greens are tender and the fish flakes when pressed lightly, about 20 minutes.

Ingredient tip Any type of salmon is delicious in this dish but the variety with the least potassium and phosphorus is Chinook salmon caught on the west coast of Canada or the US. If it is in your budget, choose only wild-caught salmon, because its quality and taste are superior.

PER SERVING Calories: 134; Total fat: 9g; Saturated fat: 2g; Cholesterol: 36mg; Sodium: 36mg; Carbohydrates: 2g; Fiber: 1g; Phosphorus: 185mg; Potassium: 298mg; Protein: 12g

SALMON LINGUINE

Serves 4 / Prep time: 15 minutes / Cook time: 15 minutes

Salmon is high in omega-3 fatty acids, making it an easy choice when you are standing at the fish counter. The human body cannot make omega-3 acids, so people have to get this nutrient in their food. Omega-3 fatty acids help build cell membranes in the brain and support the cardiovascular system in many ways. It's also linked with helping prevent cancer and reducing the impact of autoimmune diseases. Even aside from those benefits, this rich and hearty recipe truly satisfies!

½ cup ricotta cheese

¼ cup heavy (whipping) cream

Juice and zest of ½ lemon

1 tablespoon chopped fresh thyme

¼ teaspoon freshly ground black pepper

6 ounces cooked or canned salmon, broken into chunks

1 cup (2-inch pieces) blanched asparagus spears

2 cups warm cooked linguine

1. In a medium saucepan, whisk together the ricotta cheese, cream, lemon juice, lemon zest, thyme, and pepper until well blended.

2. Place the saucepan over medium heat and cook, whisking frequently, until the sauce is hot and bubbly, about 10 minutes.

3. Stir in the salmon, asparagus, and linguine, and heat for 4 additional minutes.

4. Serve.

Cooking tip To save time and dishes, you can cook the pasta and blanch the asparagus in the same pot. Cook your pasta until it is al dente and add the asparagus. Blanch for 2 minutes, and drain the vegetables and pasta in the same strainer.

PER SERVING Calories: 287; Total fat: 13g; Saturated fat: 6g; Cholesterol: 51mg; Sodium: 65mg; Carbohydrates: 25g; Fiber: 2g; Phosphorus: 235mg; Potassium: 304mg; Protein: 17g

TUNA BURGERS

Serves 4 / Prep time: 10 minutes (plus 1 hour chilling time) / Cook time: 8 minutes

Anyone who grew up in the 1980s may remember the tasteless fish burgers that showed up for dinner every once in a while and required heaps of ketchup to make them palatable. Shed your fears: these juicy, flavorful fish patties bear no resemblance to those processed ones. If you have leftover cooked fish, such as salmon or haddock, you can use that instead of the tuna, with very similar results. Serve your fish burgers with cucumber slices and maybe a spoon of homemade tartar sauce made from equal parts mayonnaise and sweet relish, with a bit of lemon juice, chopped capers, and minced onion. Serve over a lettuce leaf or a tossed green salad, if desired.

2 (6-ounce) cans water-packed tuna, drained
½ cup bread crumbs
1 scallion, white and green parts, finely chopped
1 egg, lightly beaten

1 tablespoon Low-Sodium Mayonnaise (page 70) or store-bought
1 tablespoon chopped fresh parsley
1 teaspoon Dijon mustard
1 teaspoon freshly squeezed lemon juice
2 teaspoons olive oil

1. In a large bowl, add the tuna, bread crumbs, scallion, egg, mayonnaise, parsley, mustard, and lemon juice and stir until well mixed. If the mixture is too wet to hold together, add more bread crumbs, and if it is too dry, add more mayonnaise.

2. Shape into 4 patties, and place them in the refrigerator to firm up for 1 hour.

3. In a large skillet over medium-high heat, heat the olive oil.

4. Add the tuna patties, and fry for 3 to 4 minutes on each side or until golden.

5. Serve hot.

Low-sodium tip Several ingredients in this recipe add sodium, including the bread crumbs, mayonnaise, and Dijon mustard. Using the Low-Sodium Mayonnaise (page 70) and regular mustard will cut the sodium per serving to 98 mg.

PER SERVING Calories: 190; Total fat: 6g; Saturated fat: 1g; Cholesterol: 36mg; Sodium: 159mg; Carbohydrates: 10g; Fiber: 1g; Phosphorus: 196mg; Potassium: 231mg; Protein: 22g

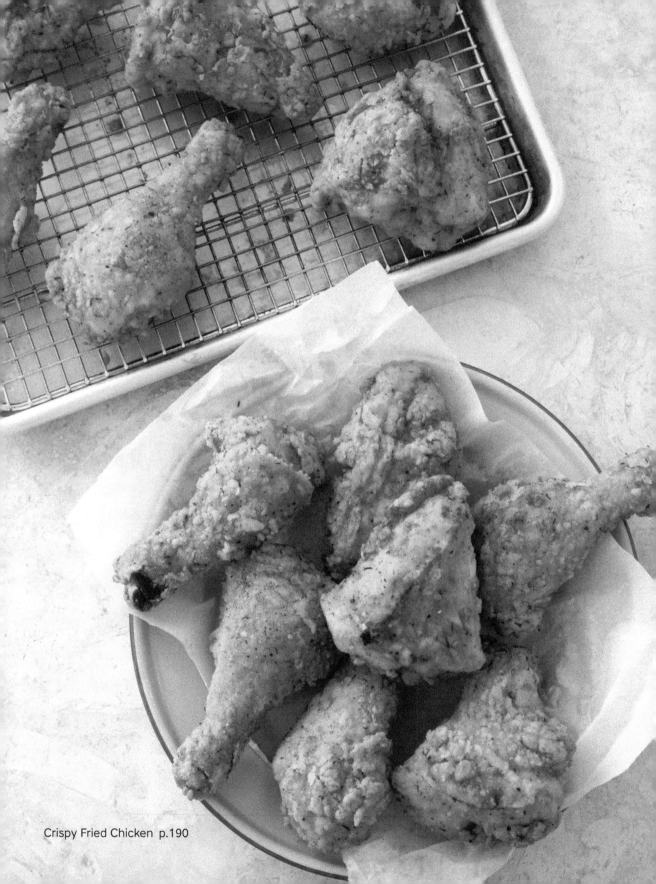

Crispy Fried Chicken p.190

12

POULTRY AND MEAT DISHES

SWEET CHICKEN STIR-FRY

Serves 4 / Prep time: 20 minutes / Cook time: 20 minutes

LOW PROTEIN LOW FAT Depending on how often you create Asian-themed meals like this colorful sweet and sour stir-fry, it might be worthwhile to purchase a wok. "Wok" is the Cantonese word for a specialty pan used to cook many Chinese dishes. These pans have curved bottoms and sloping sides that allow you to cook with very little oil and move the food from the concentrated heat spot at the bottom to cooler parts on the sides. This advantage is perfect for stir-frying, because as long as you stir, the ingredients do not overcook!

1 tablespoon low-sodium soy sauce

1 teaspoon apple cider vinegar

1 teaspoon freshly squeezed lemon juice

1 teaspoon honey

1 teaspoon cornstarch

Pinch red pepper flakes

2 teaspoons toasted sesame oil

8 ounces boneless skinless chicken breast cut into 1-inch chunks

1 cup halved fresh mushrooms

1 teaspoon minced garlic

1 red bell pepper, cut into thin strips

1 carrot, julienned

1 scallion, white and green parts, sliced

1 tablespoon toasted sesame seeds

1. In a small bowl, add the soy sauce, vinegar, lemon juice, honey, cornstarch, and red pepper flakes and whisk to mix well. Set it aside.

2. In a large skillet over medium-high heat, heat the sesame oil. Add the chicken pieces, and sauté until browned and just cooked through, about 7 minutes.

3. With a slotted spoon, remove the chicken to a plate.

4. Add the mushrooms and garlic to the skillet, and sauté until softened, about 5 minutes.

5. Stir in the bell pepper and carrot, and stir-fry until the vegetables are crisp-tender, about 5 minutes.

6. Move the vegetables to one side of the skillet, and pour the sauce in the other side.

7. Whisk the sauce until thickened and glossy, about 3 minutes.

8. Return the chicken to the skillet, and toss it in the sauce with the vegetables.

9. Serve topped with the scallion and toasted sesame seeds.

Low-sodium tip If you need to be very strict with your sodium but still want to enjoy a lovely stir-fry, you can omit the soy sauce. This will reduce the sodium per portion to about 45mg.

PER SERVING Calories: 114; Total fat: 3g; Saturated fat: 1g; Cholesterol: 32mg; Sodium: 298mg; Carbohydrates: 5g; Fiber: 1g; Phosphorus: 135mg; Potassium: 265mg; Protein: 14g

MARINATED CHICKEN

Serves 4 / Prep time: 10 minutes (plus 2 hours marinating time) / Cook time: 30 minutes

You might be reminded of goulash, a traditional Hungarian dish, when you first taste this gorgeous golden chicken. Paprika is an extremely popular spice in Hungary, used generously in many recipes. If you want to highlight this similarity in taste, serve the chicken topped with a teaspoon of light sour cream and a sprinkle of freshly chopped parsley.

½ cup chopped sweet onion

¼ cup olive oil

2 tablespoons freshly squeezed
   lemon juice

1 tablespoon chopped fresh oregano

1 teaspoon minced garlic

1 teaspoon smoked paprika

4 (3-ounce) boneless skinless
   chicken thighs

1. In a blender, add the onion, olive oil, lemon juice, oregano, garlic, and paprika and purée.

2. Pour into a large resealable plastic bag, and add the chicken thighs.

3. Press the air out of the bag, seal, and place in the refrigerator so the chicken can marinate for 2 hours, turning it several times.

4. Preheat the oven to 400°F.

5. Place the chicken in a baking dish, and discard the remaining marinade.

6. Roast the chicken until it is cooked through, about 30 minutes.

7. Serve hot.

Cooking tip Don't leave your chicken any longer than 2 hours in the marinade or you can end up doing the opposite of what you are trying to achieve. If left too long, the acid in the marinade will tighten the protein strands, which creates a tough meat rather than tender. This is true of all meats and all acidic marinades, like citrus, vinegar, or wine.

PER SERVING Calories: 154; Total fat: 8g; Saturated fat: 1g; Cholesterol: 49mg; Sodium: 55mg; Carbohydrates: 0g; Fiber: 0g; Phosphorus: 165mg; Potassium: 222mg; Protein: 19g

TUNISIAN SPICED CHICKEN

Serves 4 / Prep time: 10 minutes / Cook time: 40 minutes

LOW FAT Tunisian cooking may not be familiar to you, but it is a fusion of cuisines including French, Arabic, and Mediterranean. The cilantro in this recipe blends nicely with the other flavorings like cumin, ginger, and turmeric. Cilantro is rich in calcium, magnesium, and vitamins A, C, and K. This pungent herb can lower the risk of diabetes, heart disease, and osteoporosis; cleanse toxins from the body; and support healthy skin.

1 tablespoon olive oil

12 ounces boneless skinless
  chicken thighs

¼ small sweet onion, chopped

1 tablespoon grated peeled fresh ginger

2 teaspoons minced garlic

1 teaspoon paprika

1 teaspoon ground coriander

½ teaspoon ground cumin

¼ teaspoon ground turmeric

¼ teaspoon ground allspice

¾ cup basmati rice

1½ cups water

2 tablespoons chopped fresh cilantro

1. In a large skillet over medium-high heat, heat the olive oil.

2. Add the chicken and brown on both sides, about 6 minutes total. Transfer to a plate.

3. In the skillet, add the onion, ginger, and garlic and sauté until softened, about 3 minutes.

4. Stir in the paprika, coriander, cumin, turmeric, allspice, and rice and mix well to coat the rice with the spices.

5. Add the water and the chicken, and bring the mixture to a boil. Reduce the heat to low, cover the skillet, and simmer until the liquid is absorbed and the chicken is cooked through, about 30 minutes.

6. Garnish with the cilantro, and serve hot.

Ingredient tip Cilantro can be an acquired taste—it is an herb that people seem to either adore or avoid. If you're a fan, try growing your own in pots in the kitchen window so you always have it on hand and can clip off exactly the right amount for a recipe.

PER SERVING Calories: 265; Total fat: 7g; Saturated fat: 1g; Cholesterol: 70mg; Sodium: 74mg; Carbohydrates: 29g; Fiber: 1g; Phosphorus: 189mg; Potassium: 264mg; Protein: 19g

CLASSIC CHICKEN POT PIE

Serves 6 / Prep time: 15 minutes / Cook time: 45 minutes

LOW PROTEIN Pies usually involve completely encasing your ingredients, either sweet or savory, in pastry, so this recipe might not technically be a pie. The herbed chicken stew is covered by the crust so the calories, fat, and sodium will be half that of a two-crust pie preparation. You lose none of the delicious taste when you omit the bottom crust.

3 tablespoons unsalted butter

½ small sweet onion, chopped

2 teaspoons minced garlic

3 tablespoons all-purpose flour

1 cup sodium-free chicken stock

1 teaspoon chopped fresh thyme

Freshly ground black pepper

1 carrot, diced

½ sweet potato, peeled and diced

2 cups chopped cooked chicken breast

½ cup frozen peas

1 store-bought 9-inch pie shell

1. Preheat the oven to 425°F.

2. In a large saucepan over medium-high heat, melt the butter.

3. Add the onion and garlic, and sauté until softened, about 3 minutes.

4. Whisk in the flour to form a paste, and cook for 1 minute.

5. Whisk in the chicken stock, and cook until the sauce thickens, about 6 minutes.

6. Whisk in the thyme, and season the sauce with pepper.

7. Remove the sauce from the heat and set it aside.

8. In a medium saucepan of boiling water, add the carrot and sweet potato, and cook until tender, about 6 minutes. Drain, and add the vegetables to the sauce.

9. Add the chicken and peas to the sauce, and stir to combine. Spoon the chicken mixture into a 9-inch casserole dish.

10. Arrange the pie crust over the chicken mixture, cut off any excess around the edges, press the crust to the casserole dish to seal, and with a paring knife make a few slits in the crust to allow steam to escape.

11. Bake on a baking sheet until the crust is golden and the filling is bubbly, about 30 minutes.

Low-sodium tip The premade crust in this recipe is convenient, but it does add about 120 mg of sodium per serving. If you have a light hand with pastry, whip up your own homemade crust with little or no salt.

PER SERVING Calories: 266; Total fat: 14g; Saturated fat: 5g; Cholesterol: 55mg; Sodium: 191mg; Carbohydrates: 18g; Fiber: 1g; Phosphorus: 130mg; Potassium: 254mg; Protein: 16g

CRISPY FRIED CHICKEN

Serves 4 / Prep time: 15 minutes / Cook time: 30 minutes

LOW FAT If you are expecting battered fried chicken with this recipe, you might be disappointed—until you taste these crispy golden thighs. Since the chicken is not immersed in oil like traditional fried chicken, the calories and fat are considerably reduced without sacrificing taste. You will find that cold leftovers are tasty as well, and there's no coagulated grease to contend with, just juicy chicken.

½ cup all-purpose flour

2 eggs, beaten

½ cup Italian seasoned bread crumbs

¼ teaspoon smoked paprika

12 ounces boneless skinless
   chicken thighs

Pinch freshly ground pepper

Olive oil cooking spray

1. Preheat the oven to 350°F.
2. Place the flour on a plate, the eggs in a shallow bowl, and the bread crumbs and paprika on another plate. Line the three dishes in a row.
3. Season a piece of chicken with pepper, and dredge it first in the flour, then the egg, then the bread crumbs until the chicken is completely coated. Repeat for the remaining chicken.
4. Arrange the chicken on a baking sheet, and coat lightly with cooking spray.
5. Bake until the chicken is cooked through, browned, and crispy, about 30 minutes.
6. Serve hot.

Low-sodium tip Commercially prepared bread crumbs can be high in sodium, depending on their ingredients. The best low-sodium option is to make your own bread crumbs by pulsing stale sodium-free white bread in a food processor (or blender) to the desired consistency.

PER SERVING Calories: 246; Total fat: 7g; Saturated fat: 2g; Cholesterol: 175mg; Sodium: 206mg; Carbohydrates: 22g; Fiber: 1g; Phosphorus: 218mg; Potassium: 261mg; Protein: 23g

TANDOORI CHICKEN

Serves 4 / Prep time: 15 minutes (plus 1 hour marinating time) / Cook time: 30 minutes

LOW FAT The spice *garam masala*, used in this dish, might be unfamiliar if you do not eat much northern Indian cuisine. This spice mix is quite common in that region, and usually contains fennel, bay leaf, chile, cumin, coriander, nutmeg, and cardamom. Garam masala means "warming spice mix," accurate here because it seems to wake up the flavors of the other ingredients and warm your mouth.

6 tablespoons plain yogurt

1 tablespoon freshly squeezed lemon juice

2 teaspoons grated peeled fresh ginger

2 teaspoons garam masala

1½ teaspoons curry powder

1 teaspoon honey

1 teaspoon minced garlic

½ teaspoon paprika

Pinch cayenne pepper

4 (3-ounce) boneless skinless
   chicken breasts

1. In a medium bowl, whisk together the yogurt, lemon juice, ginger, garam masala, curry powder, honey, garlic, paprika, and cayenne pepper until well blended.

2. Add the chicken breasts to the bowl, and turn to coat. Cover the bowl and place it in the refrigerator for at least 1 hour, or up to 12 hours, to marinate.

3. Preheat the oven to 400°F.

4. Remove the chicken breasts from the marinade, and place them in a 9-by-9-inch baking dish.

5. Bake until the chicken is cooked through, turning once, about 30 minutes.

6. Serve hot.

Ingredient tip Garam masala is a unique spice blend that does not show up as a staple in many spice sections of regular grocery stores. Your best option for purchasing this wonderful fragrant product is to look for it in an Asian market. You can also make your own at home with a blend of the spices listed in the headnote.

PER SERVING Calories: 108; Total fat: 2g; Saturated fat: 1g; Cholesterol: 51mg; Sodium: 61mg; Carbohydrates: 2g; Fiber: 0g; Phosphorus: 159mg; Potassium: 220mg; Protein: 22g

CURRIED TURKEY BAKE

Serves 6 / Prep time: 15 minutes / Cook time: 30 minutes

Some dishes seem to be designed to sit in a pretty casserole dish on a potluck table at a festive local event. A never-fail casserole recipe, guaranteed to please, is a valuable addition to any recipe file. This creamy, slightly exotic dish will likely become a family favorite, and you'll be asked many times to provide the recipe if you serve it at large gatherings.

1 tablespoon olive oil, plus more for the baking dish

1 medium sweet onion, chopped

2 teaspoons minced garlic

¼ cup all-purpose flour

1 cup sodium-free chicken stock

1 cup water

½ cup heavy (whipping) cream

1 tablespoon curry powder

2 cups cauliflower florets

1 red bell pepper, diced

8 ounces cooked turkey

2 cups cooked basmati rice

1. Preheat the oven to 400°F.

2. Lightly coat a 9-by-9-inch baking dish with olive oil.

3. In a large saucepan over medium-high heat, heat 1 tablespoon of olive oil.

4. Add the onion and garlic, and sauté until softened, about 3 minutes.

5. Whisk in the flour to form a paste, and cook for 1 minute.

6. Whisk in the chicken stock, water, and cream and continue whisking until the sauce thickens, about 5 minutes.

7. Whisk in the curry powder, and remove the sauce from the heat.

8. Stir in the cauliflower, bell pepper, turkey, and rice.

9. Spoon the mixture into the prepared casserole dish. Bake until the casserole is heated through and bubbly, about 20 minutes.

10. Serve hot.

Ingredient tip Unlike cooked chicken, cooked turkey is hard to find in the store, especially a product that is not loaded with sodium. That fact makes this recipe the perfect use for leftover turkey meat after a holiday feast.

PER SERVING Calories: 265; Total fat: 13g; Saturated fat: 5g; Cholesterol: 59mg; Sodium: 108mg; Carbohydrates: 24g; Fiber: 2g; Phosphorus: 159mg; Potassium: 321mg; Protein: 15g

HONEY PORK

Serves 4 / Prep time: 10 minutes / Cook time: 12 minutes

LOW FAT The sweetness of the honey in this pork dish is countered and complemented by the presence of cayenne pepper. A little cayenne pepper goes a long way in a recipe—even a pinch can add discernible heat to a dish. Cayenne, ground from dried peppers, is packed with capsaicin, the burning element that's also an anti-inflammatory. Cayenne is also high in beta-carotene, manganese, and vitamins A, C, E, and K. Including this hot spice in your meals regularly can actually decrease the severity of cluster headaches and asthma symptoms, as well as reduce the risk of stroke and diabetes.

2 teaspoons smoked paprika

1 teaspoon dried oregano

1 teaspoon dried basil

Pinch cayenne pepper

4 (3-ounce) portions boneless pork tenderloin, cut into medallions about ½ inch thick

¼ cup honey

1. In a small bowl, stir together the paprika, oregano, basil, and cayenne pepper.

2. Rub the pork medallions generously with the spice mixture.

3. Preheat the oven to broil, and position an oven rack in the top third of the oven.

4. Place a wire rack on a baking sheet, and arrange the pork on the rack.

5. Broil the pork for 4 minutes on each side.

6. Brush the pork with the honey and broil for 2 more minutes. Turn the pork over, brush again with honey, and broil for 2 additional minutes.

7. Serve hot.

Cooking tip Honey comes in a delectable range of flavors, which depend on the type of flowers that the bees collect nectar from in their area. Try robust buckwheat honey, delicate clover honey, and other types to see which product works best.

PER SERVING Calories: 165; Total fat: 3g; Saturated fat: 1g; Cholesterol: 55mg; Sodium: 45mg; Carbohydrates: 17g; Fiber: 0g; Phosphorus: 199mg; Potassium: 331mg; Protein: 17g

PORK WITH BALSAMIC VINEGAR

Serves 4 / Prep time: 10 minutes / Cook time: 20 minutes

LOW PROTEIN Pork tenderloin can be purchased as a petite cut, or it can be several pounds in size. If you can only find the larger piece of pork, simply cut off the amount you need for this recipe, 12 ounces, and freeze the rest. Portion the pork before freezing so you can take out exactly what you need for other recipes.

4 (3-ounce) portions boneless pork tenderloin, cut into medallions about ½ inch thick

Freshly ground black pepper

¼ cup balsamic vinegar

2 teaspoons chopped fresh thyme

1 teaspoon minced garlic

¼ teaspoon red pepper flakes

1 tablespoon olive oil

1.   Preheat the oven to 400°F.

2.   Lightly season the pork with black pepper.

3.   In a small saucepan over medium heat, whisk the vinegar, thyme, garlic, and red pepper flakes.

4.   Bring the mixture to a boil, reduce the heat to low, and simmer, stirring frequently, until thick enough to coat the back of a spoon, 6 to 7 minutes.

5.   In a large ovenproof skillet over medium-high heat, add the olive oil.

6.   Sear the pork on both sides, about 2 minutes per side.

7.   Brush the pork with the balsamic vinegar glaze, and place the skillet in the oven for 4 minutes.

8.   Turn the pork over, brush the other side with the balsamic vinegar glaze, and roast for 4 minutes.

9.   Brush the pork one more time with the balsamic vinegar glaze, and serve.

Substitution tip Pork tenderloin is incredibly lean and very simple to prepare, making it a popular choice for home cooks. You can also use center cut chops or bone-in chops if you prefer. The bone-in pork will take slightly longer to cook, 3 to 5 minutes more.

PER SERVING Calories: 145; Total fat: 6g; Saturated fat: 1g; Cholesterol: 55mg; Sodium: 47mg; Carbohydrates: 3g; Fiber: 0g; Phosphorus: 207mg; Potassium: 338mg; Protein: 17g

PORK WITH BROWN SUGAR RUB

Serves 4 / Prep time: 10 minutes (plus 1 hour chilling time) / Cook time: 25 minutes

LOW FAT Chili powder has a very strong flavor that often overpowers other spices and herbs in a recipe. The addition of nutty, slightly citrusy cumin mellows the chili influence and allows for a more complex-tasting rub. Cumin is a fine source of iron, manganese, and calcium. This assertive spice boosts the immune system, improves the capacity of hemoglobin to carry oxygen, and reduces the risk of cancer. And not surprisingly, all that spice adds up to a wildly tasty dish!

1 tablespoon brown sugar

1 teaspoon chili powder

½ teaspoon ground cumin

½ teaspoon garlic powder

½ teaspoon smoked paprika

⅛ teaspoon ground allspice

4 (3-ounce) portions boneless pork tenderloin, cut into medallions about ½ inch thick

1 tablespoon olive oil

1. In a small bowl, mix together the brown sugar, chili powder, cumin, garlic powder, paprika, and allspice until well blended.

2. Rub the pork generously all over with the spice mix, and set in the refrigerator for 1 hour.

3. Preheat the oven to 400°F.

4. In a large ovenproof skillet over medium-high heat, heat the olive oil.

5. Sear the pork for 4 minutes per side, then place the skillet in the oven.

6. Roast the pork until just cooked through, about 10 minutes.

7. Serve.

Ingredient tip Smoked paprika is different from regular or sweet paprika; they each have a specific flavor and applications. Smoked paprika is usually created from Spanish pimentos that are dried and smoked over a fire to create that distinctive rich taste. You can experiment with mild spice all the way to picante until you discover your favorite.

PER SERVING Calories: 135; Total fat: 6g; Saturated fat: 1g; Cholesterol: 55mg; Sodium: 44mg; Carbohydrates: 1g; Fiber: 0g; Phosphorus: 211mg; Potassium: 334mg; Protein: 17g

GINGER SPICED LAMB CHOPS

Serves 4 / Prep time: 15 minutes (plus 1 hour marinating time) / Cook time: 8 minutes

Lamb is a reasonable choice for those who want to include meat in their diet but are watching their potassium and phosphorus. Lamb is lower in these minerals than beef or pork, and is quite close to chicken, in the same portion size. Look for organic lamb that is grass-fed, because these animals have higher levels of omega-3 fatty acids than those that are factory farmed.

2 tablespoons olive oil

1 tablespoon low-sodium soy sauce

1 tablespoon grated peeled fresh ginger

1 teaspoon minced garlic

½ teaspoon chipotle chile powder

Pinch freshly ground black pepper

4 (3-ounce) lamb chops

1 tablespoon chopped fresh cilantro

1. In a medium bowl, stir together the olive oil, soy sauce, ginger, garlic, chipotle chile powder, and pepper.

2. Add the lamb chops, and turn to coat.

3. Place the bowl in the refrigerator and marinate the chops, turning several times, for 1 hour.

4. Preheat the oven to broil, and set one of the racks in the upper third of the oven.

5. Place a wire rack in a baking sheet, and arrange the chops on the rack.

6. Broil, turning once, until the chops are browned and cooked to medium doneness, about 8 minutes total.

7. Serve sprinkled with the cilantro.

Low-sodium tip Using blackstrap molasses in the place of soy sauce can give the marinade an interesting smoky flavor, and it only has 7 mg of sodium per tablespoon. Though it's not at all salty, you might enjoy the different taste experience.

PER SERVING Calories: 146; Total fat: 8g; Saturated fat: 2g; Cholesterol: 54mg; Sodium: 306mg; Carbohydrates: 1g; Fiber: 0g; Phosphorus: 177mg; Potassium: 298mg; Protein: 18g

ITALIAN STYLE MEATBALLS

Serves 4 / Prep time: 15 minutes / Cook time: 35 minutes

Meatballs are fun to eat and so easy to make, you will have no excuse not to have them sitting on your table at least once a week. This base recipe can be spiced up any way you want with herbs, sauces, and spices. Meatballs that are Asian-themed, Tex-Mex, Swedish, or tossed in a sweet barbecue sauce all work, so double up the recipe and experiment with something different every time.

Olive oil cooking spray

12 ounces lean ground beef

1 egg

2 tablespoons bread crumbs

2 tablespoons grated Parmesan cheese

1 tablespoon chopped fresh parsley

1 teaspoon minced garlic

½ teaspoon Dijon mustard

Pinch freshly ground black pepper

1. Preheat the oven to 350°F.

2. Lightly coat a baking sheet with cooking spray.

3. In a large bowl, mix together the beef, egg, bread crumbs, Parmesan cheese, parsley, garlic, mustard, and pepper.

4. Form the meat mixture into small (1-inch) meatballs, and arrange them on the prepared baking sheet.

5. Bake until browned, turning several times, about 35 minutes.

6. Serve hot.

Low-sodium tip Dijon mustard adds a unique flavor to any dish, but it has about 115 mg of sodium per teaspoon. If you want to reduce the sodium in this recipe to under 100 mg per serving, use ¼ teaspoon dried mustard instead.

PER SERVING Calories: 159; Total fat: 6g; Saturated fat: 3g; Cholesterol: 107mg; Sodium: 143mg; Carbohydrates: 3g; Fiber: 0g; Phosphorus: 206mg; Potassium: 311mg; Protein: 21g

CAULIFLOWER-TOPPED SHEPHERD'S PIE

Serves 6 / Prep time: 15 minutes / Cook time: 40 minutes

LOW FAT Cauliflower is not just a fluffy delicious topping for this dish—it is also a nutrient-packed, kidney-friendly treat. Cauliflower is high in fiber, vitamin C, and folate as well as antioxidants like glucosinolates, which can help detoxify the liver. Cauliflower also contains a sulfur-containing compound called sulforaphane, linked to improved blood pressure and kidney health.

½ head cauliflower, cut into florets

2 tablespoons unsalted butter,
   at room temperature

12 ounces extra-lean ground beef

½ small sweet onion, diced

2 teaspoons minced garlic

2 medium tomatoes, diced

1 carrot, diced and parboiled until
   fork-tender

1 teaspoon chopped thyme

¼ teaspoon freshly ground black pepper

1. Preheat the oven to 375°F.

2. Place a large saucepan filled with water over medium-high heat, and bring to a boil.

3. Add the cauliflower, and blanch until tender, about 6 minutes.

4. Drain the cauliflower and mash with the butter until fluffy. Set it aside.

5. In a large skillet over medium-high heat, brown the beef, about 6 minutes.

6. Add the onion and garlic, and sauté until softened, about 3 minutes.

7. Stir in the tomatoes, carrot, and thyme.

8. Season with the pepper. Transfer the beef mixture to a 9-by-9-inch baking dish.

9. Top with the mashed cauliflower, and bake until bubbly, about 25 minutes.

10. Serve hot.

Substitution tip Cauliflower is a substitution of the traditional topping of fluffy mashed potatoes. You can also try mashed sweet potatoes in a thin layer, or mashed celeriac for a different taste. These add more potassium than cauliflower, so watch your daily totals.

PER SERVING Calories: 128; Total fat: 7g; Saturated fat: 4g; Cholesterol: 45mg; Sodium: 52mg; Carbohydrates: 4g; Fiber: 1g; Phosphorus: 130mg; Potassium: 341mg; Protein: 13g

SALISBURY STEAK

Serves 4 / Prep time: 15 minutes / Cook time: 25 minutes

Salisbury steak was introduced in about 1897 as a component of a low-carb diet advocated by American physician Dr. J. H. Salisbury, and it's still popular today. This dish is often made with a 3:1 beef-to-pork ratio. This version is closer to the Japanese hamburg, which includes chopped onion, egg, and seasonings.

12 ounces lean ground beef

1 small sweet onion, finely chopped

½ red bell pepper, seeded and
   finely chopped

1 teaspoon minced garlic

1 egg, beaten

½ teaspoon chopped fresh thyme

¼ teaspoon freshly ground black pepper

1 teaspoon olive oil

½ cup sodium-free beef stock, divided

1 tablespoon cornstarch

1. In a medium bowl, mix together the beef, onion, bell pepper, garlic, egg, thyme, and pepper.

2. Form the meat mixture into 4 equal patties about ½ inch thick.

3. In a medium skillet over medium-high heat, heat the olive oil. Brown the patties on both sides, about 6 minutes total.

4. Add ¼ cup of stock to the skillet and simmer for 15 minutes, turning the patties once.

5. Remove the patties to a plate, cover, and set aside.

6. Whisk the cornstarch into the remaining ¼ cup of stock, and add the mixture to the skillet.

7. Simmer, whisking, until the sauce thickens to a gravy consistency.

8. Serve the patties topped with the sauce.

Substitution tip If you have the time and inclination, consider making your own beef stock from nicely browned bones, so you can control the additives. Homemade stock can be stored in sealed containers in the freezer for up to 2 months.

PER SERVING Calories: 153; Total fat: 7g; Saturated fat: 2g; Cholesterol: 105mg; Sodium: 117mg; Carbohydrates: 2g; Fiber: 0g; Phosphorus: 193mg; Potassium: 361mg; Protein: 20g

STUFFED BELL PEPPERS

Serves 4 / Prep time: 15 minutes / Cook time: 45 minutes

LOW PROTEIN LOW FAT The red bell peppers featured in this recipe are a fabulous choice to support kidney health, for many reasons. This sweet vegetable is very low in potassium, and is high in vitamins A, C, and B_6, as well as fiber and the antioxidant called lycopene.

Olive oil, for the baking dish

4 red bell peppers, tops removed, seeded

8 ounces lean ground beef

½ small sweet onion, finely chopped

1 celery stalk, finely chopped

1 teaspoon minced garlic

½ cup cooked white rice

1 teaspoon chopped fresh oregano

½ teaspoon chopped fresh thyme

Freshly ground black pepper

2 tablespoons crumbled feta cheese

1. Preheat the oven to 350°F.

2. Lightly oil a 9-by-9-inch baking dish, and place the peppers in, hollow-side up.

3. In a large skillet over medium-high heat, add the ground beef, and brown for about 10 minutes.

4. Stir in the onion, celery, and garlic, and sauté until the vegetables are softened, about 3 minutes.

5. Stir in the rice, oregano, and thyme.

6. Season the filling with pepper, and remove from the heat.

7. Spoon the filling into the 4 peppers, dividing it evenly, and sprinkle with the feta cheese.

8. Bake the peppers until tender and the filling is heated through, about 30 minutes.

9. Serve hot.

Substitution tip Pork, chicken, turkey, and even barley can all take the place of the beef in this recipe. Substitute 1 cup of uncooked barley for the 12 ounces of ground meat, and prepare the bell peppers as directed.

PER SERVING Calories: 152; Total fat: 5g; Saturated fat: 3g; Cholesterol: 42mg; Sodium: 139mg; Carbohydrates: 11g; Fiber: 2g; Phosphorus: 174mg; Potassium: 373mg; Protein: 15g

HOMESTYLE HAMBURGERS

Serves 4 / Prep time: 15 minutes / Cook time: 15 minutes

Nothing says summer quite like sizzling hamburgers right off the barbecue. So if you have a barbecue, grill these patties instead of using a skillet. The timing is similar, and you'll add a delightful charred taste to the meat. Serve your hamburgers with favorite toppings, either on a bun or a leaf of lettuce, depending on your dietary needs.

12 ounces lean ground beef

½ cup chopped sweet onion

1 teaspoon minced fresh garlic

1 teaspoon Dijon mustard

½ teaspoon chopped fresh thyme

Pinch freshly ground black pepper

1 tablespoon olive oil

1. In a large bowl, mix together the beef, onion, garlic, mustard, thyme, and pepper until well combined.

2. Divide the meat mixture into 4 equal balls, and form into ½-inch-thick patties.

3. In a large skillet over medium-high heat, heat the olive oil.

4. Pan-fry the burgers until they are cooked through and browned, about 6 minutes per side.

5. Serve hot.

Cooking tip Raw hamburger patties freeze very well when tightly wrapped, so double up the recipe and stock up for a future meal. Place a piece of parchment paper between the patties so they are easy to separate, and cook them right from frozen.

PER SERVING Calories: 150; Total fat: 8g; Saturated fat: 2g; Cholesterol: 52mg; Sodium: 70mg; Carbohydrates: 1g; Fiber: 0g; Phosphorus: 161mg; Potassium: 298mg; Protein: 18g

STEAK WITH CREAMY MUSTARD SAUCE

Serves 4 / Prep time: 10 minutes / Cook time: 8 minutes

LOW FAT It doesn't take much to make a good sirloin steak—it's delicious sprinkled with a little spice and tossed on a hot grill. This recipe leverages the juicy goodness of this cut of meat with a savory mustard-base sauce. Grainy mustard is just like regular mustard, except the mustard seeds are not puréed into the other ingredients to create a smooth condiment. Mustard seeds are a fabulous source of omega-3 fatty acids, magnesium, and selenium. They can help lower blood pressure, reduce the risk of cancer and cardiovascular disease, and decrease the severity of migraines.

2 tablespoons grainy mustard

1 tablespoon apple cider vinegar

1 tablespoon honey

1 teaspoon minced garlic

12 ounces sirloin steak

Pinch freshly ground black pepper

1. In a small bowl, stir together the mustard, vinegar, honey, and garlic.

2. Lightly season the steak with pepper.

3. Baste the steak generously with the mustard sauce on both sides, and let it stand for 15 minutes at room temperature.

4. Preheat the oven to broil, and set a rack in the top third of the oven.

5. Place a wire rack in a baking sheet, and arrange the steak on the rack.

6. Broil the steak, turning once and basting again, until the steak is browned and cooked to medium doneness, about 8 minutes total.

7. Serve hot.

Cooking tip The best way to cook steaks is on a hot barbecue, so if you have one, by all means fire it up for this dish. Grill the meat, basting with the sauce between flips, until desired doneness, about 8 minutes total.

PER SERVING Calories: 136; Total fat: 3g; Saturated fat: 1g; Cholesterol: 39mg; Sodium: 134mg; Carbohydrates: 5g; Fiber: 0g; Phosphorus: 182mg; Potassium: 306mg; Protein: 19g

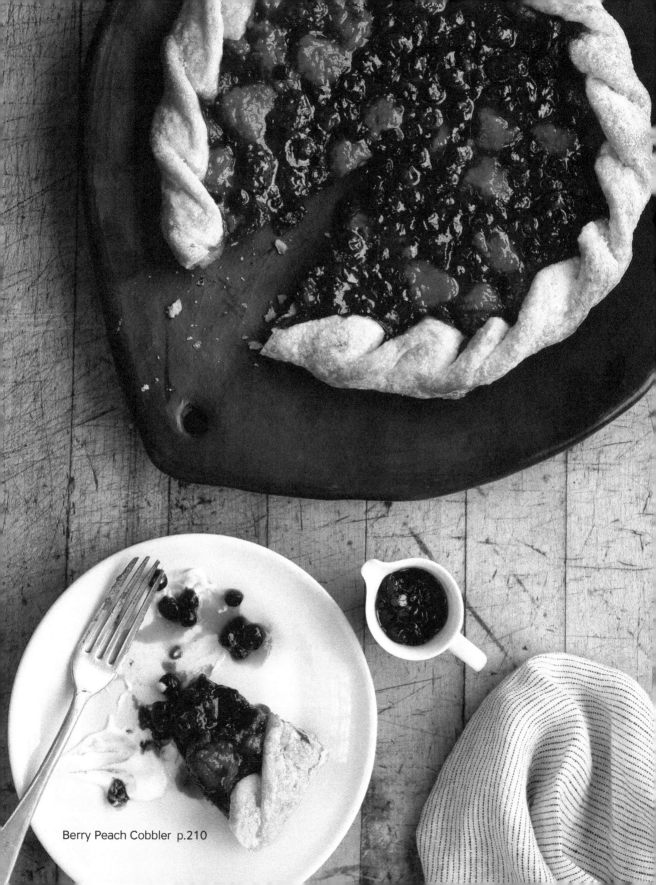

Berry Peach Cobbler p.210

13

DESSERTS

POACHED PEARS

Serves 4 / Prep time: 15 minutes / Cook time: 30 minutes

LOW PROTEIN LOW FAT Homemade poached pears are so elegant, they seem like you spent hours in the kitchen making them. The challenge in making this delectable dish is the importance of carefully peeling the pears while keeping the smooth surface of the fruit. Every little nick shows up when the pears are poached because the color of the nicked flesh is darker. If you are not as concerned with the presentation, then peel with abandon!

4 cups water

2 cups apple juice

1 cup sugar

4 pears, peeled with the stem left on

1 vanilla bean, split and seeded

1. In a large saucepan over medium heat, add the water, apple juice, and sugar. Stir the mixture until the sugar is completely dissolved, then simmer for 5 minutes.

2. Add the pears and vanilla bean and seeds to the simmering liquid, and cover the saucepan.

3. Simmer the pears, turning several times, until the pears are very tender, about 20 minutes.

4. Carefully remove the pears from the liquid with a slotted spoon, and arrange on a plate. Serve warm or cooled.

Cooking tip Recipes usually require ripe fruit in order to get the best flavor in the finished dish. In the case of poached pears, seek out pears that are a hint green so they will hold up well in the simmering process.

PER SERVING Calories: 148; Total fat: 0g; Saturated fat: 0g; Cholesterol: 0mg; Sodium: 3mg; Carbohydrates: 39g; Fiber: 5g; Phosphorus: 18mg; Potassium: 198mg; Protein: 1g

BAKED VANILLA PUDDING

Serves 4 / Prep time: 10 minutes (plus cooling time) / Cook time: 45 minutes

LOW PROTEIN LOW FAT Pudding is a childhood comfort food. Maybe you were served this when you were not feeling good and needed a pick-me-up. The best part of this already sublime vanilla pudding recipe is that you can serve it in many different ways. Try it with fresh fruit, crushed cookie pieces, a drizzle of honey, or even baked into a pie shell for a truly memorable dessert.

2 cups Homemade Rice Milk (page 80; or use unsweetened store-bought)

4 egg yolks

⅓ cup sugar

1 teaspoon vanilla extract

1. Preheat the oven to 350°F.

2. Place four (4-ounce) ramekins in a 9-by-9-inch baking pan, and pour water into the pan so it comes halfway up the sides of the ramekins.

3. In a large bowl, add the rice milk, egg yolks, sugar, and vanilla and whisk well.

4. Pour the egg mixture into the ramekins, dividing it evenly, and cover the baking dish with foil.

5. Bake the puddings until they are set, about 45 minutes.

6. Let the ramekins cool in the water, then chill them in the refrigerator. Serve cold.

Ingredient tip When purchasing vanilla beans, you can choose from two kinds: Madagascar Bourbon vanilla beans, which have a strong, assertive vanilla flavor; or Tahitian vanilla beans, which are more fruity, floral, and sweet.

PER SERVING Calories: 177; Total fat: 5g; Saturated fat: 2g; Cholesterol: 210mg; Sodium: 48mg; Carbohydrates: 29g; Fiber: 0g; Phosphorus: 66mg; Potassium: 20mg; Protein: 3g

LEMON MOUSSE

Serves 6 / Prep time: 35 minutes (plus cooling time) / Cook time: 5 minutes

LOW PROTEIN This dessert takes some time and effort to create, but you will be pleased with the results, especially if you are making it for cherished guests. A hand mixer will make the job much easier, though a determined cook can use a whisk for all stages of preparation. Lay a wet cloth on your counter when whisking the whipped cream and egg whites, so the bowls don't slip.

4 eggs, separated

½ cup sugar

¼ cup freshly squeezed lemon juice

1 tablespoon freshly grated lemon zest

1 teaspoon vanilla extract

½ cup heavy cream, whipped to stiff peaks

1. In a large bowl, beat the egg yolks until very thick and pale yellow.

2. Fold in the sugar by tablespoons, beating well after each addition, and scraping down the sides of the bowl.

3. Beat in the lemon juice and lemon zest.

4. Heat a large saucepan with about 2 inches of water to a boil.

5. Reduce the heat to low so the water is simmering. Place the bowl with the egg yolk mixture into the water.

6. Whisk the egg mixture until it thickens and coats the back of a spoon, about 5 minutes. Remove the bowl from the heat, and cool to room temperature.

7. Fold the whipped cream gently into the egg yolk mixture to lighten it, keeping as much volume as possible.

8. In another large bowl, beat the egg whites until they form stiff peaks.

9. Fold the egg whites into the lemon mousse carefully.

10. Spoon the lemon mousse into individual bowls and serve.

Ingredient tip If you are concerned about using raw egg whites, you can purchase pasteurized eggs, which reduce the risk of salmonella to almost zero. You can also leave the whipped egg whites out altogether, but the mousse won't be as light.

PER SERVING Calories: 185; Total fat: 11g; Saturated fat: 6g; Cholesterol: 168mg; Sodium: 54mg; Carbohydrates: 18g; Fiber: 0g; Phosphorus: 76mg; Potassium: 74mg; Protein: 5g

BLUEBERRY RASPBERRY GALETTE

Serves 8 / Prep time: 20 minutes / Cook time: 30 minutes

LOW PROTEIN **LOW FAT** Fruit pies do not need to be elaborate with braided or complicated lattice crusts topping a bevy of ingredients. A couple handfuls of fresh, juicy fruit and a simple folded crust can look elegant and taste glorious. Any fruit will do in a simple pie—just be sure to stir in some cornstarch so the juices don't create a soggy crust.

2 cups fresh blueberries

1 cup fresh raspberries

½ cup sugar

1 tablespoon cornstarch

¼ teaspoon ground nutmeg

1 (9-inch) prepared, flat, unbaked piecrust

1 egg, beaten

1. Preheat the oven to 400°F.

2. Line a baking sheet with parchment paper.

3. In a large bowl, add the blueberries, raspberries, sugar, cornstarch, and nutmeg and toss gently to mix together.

4. Lay the piecrust on the parchment paper in the prepared pan, and pour the berry mixture into the center.

5. Spread out the berries, leaving about 1½ inches of bare crust around the edges.

6. Brush the bare crust with the egg. Fold the edges of the crust back over the filling, pressing lightly so the overlapping pastry folds stick together.

7. Bake the galette until the crust is golden and crisp and the berries are bubbling, about 30 minutes.

8. Serve.

Cooking tip This style of freeform crust is easy to work with, but if you prefer a more traditional presentation, you can arrange the crust and filling in a pie pan instead. The pie will take about the same time to cook.

PER SERVING Calories: 196; Total fat: 5g; Saturated fat: 1g; Cholesterol: 0mg; Sodium: 56mg; Carbohydrates: 45g; Fiber: 2g; Phosphorus: 19mg; Potassium: 144mg; Protein: 4g

BERRY PEACH COBBLER

Serves 8 / Prep time: 15 minutes / Cook time: 35 minutes

LOW PROTEIN Oats can be consumed on a renal diet even though they have more potassium than some other grains. Oats offer many nutrients that are beneficial for people who have kidney disease, such as vitamin B_6 and iron, which can help prevent kidney stones. Many people with kidney issues also have an iron deficiency, so any food that can replenish this mineral is a good thing.

4 tablespoons melted unsalted butter,
   plus more for the baking dish
2 cups mixed fresh berries
2 peaches, peeled, pitted, and sliced
¼ cup sugar
1 tablespoon cornstarch

½ teaspoon ground nutmeg
¾ cup almond meal
¼ cup rolled oats
1 teaspoon Phosphorus-Free Baking
   Powder (page 65)

1. Preheat the oven to 350°F.

2. Lightly coat a 9-by-9-inch baking dish with melted butter.

3. In a medium bowl, toss together the berries, peaches, sugar, cornstarch, and nutmeg.

4. Transfer the fruit mixture to the baking dish, and spread it out evenly.

5. In a medium bowl, use a fork to stir together the almond meal, oats, and baking powder until well blended. Stir in 4 tablespoons of melted butter, tossing to form coarse crumbs.

6. Top the fruit mixture evenly with the oat mixture.

7. Bake the cobbler until bubbly and golden brown, about 35 minutes. Serve warm or cold.

Ingredient tip Almond meal, also known as almond flour, comes in varying consistencies depending on how long the nuts were processed. This recipe is best with a slightly coarser texture. You can make your own, but take care not to pulse too much with the food processor (or blender), or you'll produce almond butter.

PER SERVING Calories: 158; Total fat: 9g; Saturated fat: 4g; Cholesterol: 15mg; Sodium: 42mg; Carbohydrates: 18g; Fiber: 2g; Phosphorus: 69mg; Potassium: 199mg; Protein: 3g

LEMON CAKE

Serves 8 / Prep time: 20 minutes / Cook time: 1 hour

LOW PROTEIN Many ingredients that go into traditional cake recipes are high in potassium and phosphorus, which can limit the type of desserts that people with kidney issues can enjoy on special occasions. This cake is prepared in a loaf pan, and the serving size is a slice about 1-inch thick. If you choose a smaller piece of cake, you can add a tablespoon of whipped cream topping and fresh fruit without compromising your diet.

½ cup unsalted butter, plus more
   for the pan

1 cup all-purpose flour, plus more
   for the pan

½ cup sugar

4 eggs

⅓ cup freshly squeezed lemon juice

1 teaspoon vanilla extract

½ teaspoon Phosphorus-Free Baking
   Powder (page 65)

2 tablespoons freshly grated lemon zest

1. Preheat the oven to 350°F.

2. Lightly coat an 8-by-4-inch loaf pan with butter and dust with flour.

3. In a large bowl, beat together ½ cup of butter and the sugar until fluffy.

4. Beat in the eggs one at a time, scraping down the sides of the bowl after each addition. Beat in the lemon juice and vanilla.

5. In a small bowl, whisk together 1 cup of flour, the baking powder, and lemon zest until well mixed. Add the flour mixture to the butter mixture and whisk until blended.

6. Spoon the batter into the prepared pan. Bake until the cake springs back when touched, about 1 hour. Cool completely and serve.

Cooking tip Scrub lemons thoroughly before zesting them because these fruits are often coated in wax to protect them during transportation. Scrubbing them will prevent transferring the wax to your cake.

PER SERVING Calories: 245; Total fat: 14g; Saturated fat: 8g; Cholesterol: 136mg; Sodium: 37mg; Carbohydrates: 25g; Fiber: 0g; Phosphorus: 69mg; Potassium: 78mg; Protein: 5g

SPICED GINGERBREAD

Serves 8 / Prep time: 15 minutes (plus cooling time) / Cook time: 45 minutes

LOW PROTEIN Even the scant amount of allspice in this yummy gingerbread packs a fragrant punch and adds a warm element to the flavor combination. The name "allspice" originated in the 1600s when an Englishman thought this ground dried fruit was a blend of other spices. Allspice is high in calcium, manganese, iron, zinc, and vitamin C.

¾ cup unsalted butter, at room temperature, plus more for the pan

1¼ cups all-purpose flour, plus more for the pan

¾ cup sugar

3 eggs

2 teaspoons vanilla extract

1 teaspoon ground ginger

½ teaspoon ground cinnamon

½ teaspoon Phosphorus-Free Baking Powder (page 65)

¼ teaspoon ground allspice

1. Preheat the oven to 350°F.

2. Lightly coat an 8-by-4-inch loaf pan with butter and dust with flour.

3. In a large bowl, beat together ¾ cup of butter and the sugar until light and fluffy.

4. Add the eggs, one at a time, beating well after each addition, and scraping down the sides of the bowl.

5. Beat in the vanilla.

6. In a medium bowl, whisk together 1¼ cups of flour, the ginger, cinnamon, baking powder, and allspice.

7. Add the flour mixture to the egg mixture, and stir to blend well.

8. Spoon the batter into the loaf pan and spread it out evenly. Bake until golden brown and a toothpick inserted near the center comes out clean, about 45 minutes.

9. Cool the gingerbread for 10 minutes before removing from the pan to a wire rack to cool completely.

10. Serve warm or chilled.

Cooking tip This recipe can also be used to make pretty cupcakes for a fall birthday party treat or Christmas bake sale item. Simply frost them with a swirl of sweet cream cheese icing and a pinch of cinnamon.

PER SERVING Calories: 326; Total fat: 19g; Saturated fat: 12g; Cholesterol: 125mg; Sodium: 29mg; Carbohydrates: 34g; Fiber: 1g; Phosphorus: 62mg; Potassium: 68mg; Protein: 5g

SPICED APPLE CAKE

Serves 12 / Prep time: 15 minutes / Cook time: 60 minutes

LOW PROTEIN **LOW FAT** Apples are one of the fruits recommended on a kidney-friendly diet because they are low in potassium and naturally cleanse the body. Apples are a fabulous source of fiber, specifically pectin, a soluble fiber that can prevent blood sugar spikes and can help to lower cholesterol. Apples also help fight cancer and support cardiovascular health because they are high in the antioxidant quercetin.

¼ cup unsalted butter, at room temperature, plus more for the baking dish

2 apples, peeled, cored, and diced

2 tablespoons freshly squeezed lemon juice

½ cup sugar

¼ cup honey

1 egg

2 cups all-purpose flour

1 teaspoon Phosphorus-Free Baking Powder (page 65)

1 teaspoon ground cinnamon

½ teaspoon baking soda

¼ teaspoon ground nutmeg

1. Preheat the oven to 350°F.

2. Lightly coat a 9-by-9-inch baking dish with butter.

3. In a large bowl, toss the apples with the lemon juice.

4. In another large bowl, beat together ¼ cup of butter, the sugar, and honey until fluffy.

5. Beat in the egg, scraping down the sides of the bowl.

6. In a medium bowl, whisk together the flour, baking powder, cinnamon, baking soda, and nutmeg.

7. Add the butter mixture to the flour mixture, and stir into combine.

8. Stir in the apples. Pour the batter to the prepared baking dish.

9. Bake until golden brown and a knife inserted in the center comes out clean, about 60 minutes.

10. Serve warm or cold.

Ingredient tip Nutmeg is a common spice, easily found in the spice section of the supermarket. For a more intense, freshly ground flavor, source out the whole nutmeg seed, sold in spice bottles, and grate your own as needed. You can buy a micrograter for this purpose.

PER SERVING Calories: 274; Total fat: 7g; Saturated fat: 4g; Cholesterol: 42mg; Sodium: 11mg; Carbohydrates: 49g; Fiber: 2g; Phosphorus: 52mg; Potassium: 107mg; Protein: 4g

CREAM CHEESE POUND CAKE

Serves 16 / Prep time: 15 minutes (plus 15 minutes cooling time) / Cook time: 1 hour and 15 minutes

LOW PROTEIN There is no baking soda or baking powder in this recipe, which may seem surprising since leaveners are usually a crucial part of baking. This is a heavier cake, so that airiness is not needed to create a full and fabulous texture and presentation. Omitting the leavening ingredients also allows the use of the cream cheese in the recipe, because leaveners usually contain lots of potassium and phosphorus.

½ cup unsalted butter, at room temperature, plus more for the pan

3 cups sifted all-purpose flour, plus more for the pan

1 cup plain cream cheese, at room temperature

2½ cups sugar

6 eggs

1 cup Homemade Rice Milk (page 80; or use unsweetened store-bought)

1 teaspoon vanilla extract

1. Preheat the oven to 325°F.
2. Lightly coat a Bundt pan with butter and dust with flour.
3. In a large bowl, beat together the cream cheese, ½ cup of butter, and the sugar until fluffy.
4. Beat in each egg, one at a time, scraping down the sides of the bowl.
5. Add the 3 cups of flour and the rice milk in five alternating steps, starting and ending with the flour. Stir in the vanilla until well blended.
6. Transfer the batter to the prepared Bundt pan. Bake until a knife inserted in the center comes out clean, about 1 hour and 15 minutes.
7. Cool the cake for 15 minutes, then remove from the pan and cool completely on a wire rack. Serve.

Substitution tip Cream cheese adds a delightful tanginess to this dessert, but it can be replaced by another soft cheese if you want to experiment. Mascarpone, Neufchâtel, and soft goat cheese all work well in the same amount as the cream cheese.

PER SERVING Calories: 273; Total fat: 6g; Saturated fat: 4g; Cholesterol: 17mg; Sodium: 100mg; Carbohydrates: 50g; Fiber: 1g; Phosphorus: 100mg; Potassium: 67mg; Protein: 5g

CREAMSICLE CHEESECAKE

Serves 8 / Prep time: 20 minutes (plus 3 hours chilling time)

LOW PROTEIN The sweetness of the oranges blends with the tanginess of the cream cheese in this perfectly balanced dessert. Oranges are an excellent source of vitamins C and A, folate, calcium, and a phytonutrient called limonoid. Oranges reduce the risk of cancer, lower cholesterol, boost the immune system, and even fight the common cold. Make sure to scrub your orange thoroughly before zesting it to remove any unwanted contaminants.

1 envelope powdered gelatin

¼ cup cold water

14 ounces plain cream cheese, at room temperature

3 tablespoons honey

Juice and zest of ½ orange

1 teaspoon vanilla extract

1 cup heavy cream, whipped to stiff peaks

1. Line the bottom of a springform pan with parchment paper.

2. In a small bowl, sprinkle the gelatin over the cold water and let it stand for 10 minutes.

3. In a large bowl, beat together the cream cheese, honey, orange juice, orange zest, and vanilla until smooth.

4. Beat the gelatin into the cream cheese mixture until well blended.

5. Gently fold the whipped cream into the cream cheese mixture, keeping as much volume as possible.

6. Transfer the cheesecake mixture to the springform pan, and chill in the refrigerator until firm, about 3 hours.

7. Run a knife around the edges of the pan and remove the ring.

8. Slice and serve.

Low-sodium tip The sodium level in this recipe isn't staggeringly high, but don't substitute fat-free cream cheese for regular to cut calories. Fat-free cream cheese has 197 mg of sodium per ounce, compared to regular cream cheese with 90 mg for the same amount.

PER SERVING Calories: 300; Total fat: 28g; Saturated fat: 16g; Cholesterol: 95mg; Sodium: 171mg; Carbohydrates: 10g; Fiber: 0g; Phosphorus: 72mg; Potassium: 105mg; Protein: 4g

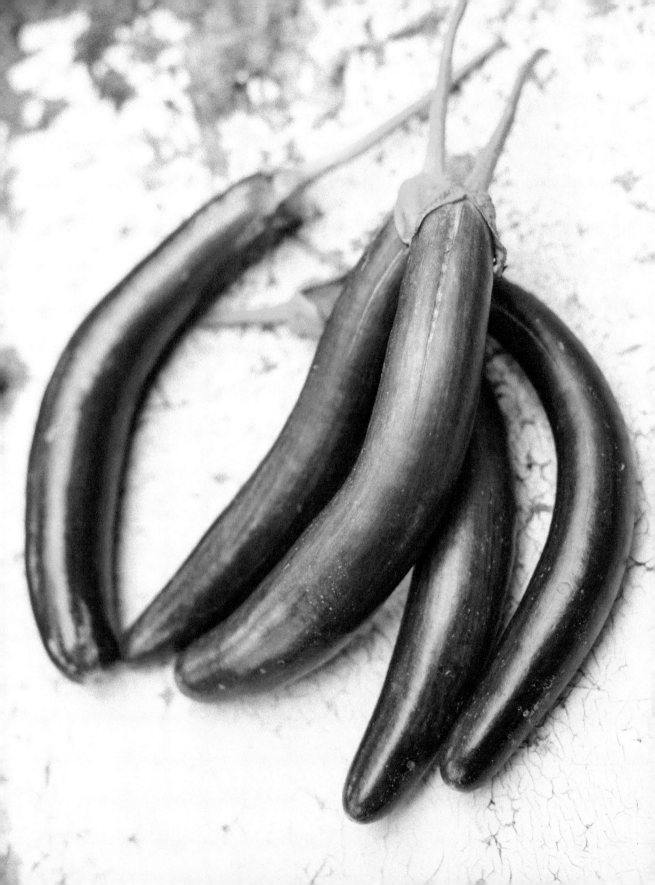

MEASUREMENT CONVERSIONS

Volume Equivalents (Liquid)

US STANDARD	US STANDARD (OUNCES)	METRIC (APPROXIMATE)
2 tablespoons	1 fl. oz.	30 mL
¼ cup	2 fl. oz.	60 mL
½ cup	4 fl. oz.	120 mL
1 cup	8 fl. oz.	240 mL
1½ cups	12 fl. oz.	355 mL
2 cups or 1 pint	16 fl. oz.	475 mL
4 cups or 1 quart	32 fl. oz.	1 L
1 gallon	128 fl. oz.	4 L

Oven Temperatures

FAHRENHEIT	CELSIUS (APPROXIMATE)
250°F	120°C
300°F	150°C
325°F	165°C
350°F	180°C
375°F	190°C
400°F	200°C
425°F	220°C
450°F	230°C

Volume Equivalents (Dry)

US STANDARD	METRIC (APPROXIMATE)
⅛ teaspoon	0.5 mL
¼ teaspoon	1 mL
½ teaspoon	2 mL
¾ teaspoon	4 mL
1 teaspoon	5 mL
1 tablespoon	15 mL
¼ cup	59 mL
⅓ cup	79 mL
½ cup	118 mL
⅔ cup	156 mL
¾ cup	177 mL
1 cup	235 mL
2 cups or 1 pint	475 mL
3 cups	700 mL
4 cups or 1 quart	1 L

Weight Equivalents

US STANDARD	METRIC (APPROXIMATE)
½ ounce	15 g
1 ounce	30 g
2 ounces	60 g
4 ounces	115 g
8 ounces	225 g
12 ounces	340 g
16 ounces or 1 pound	455 g

THE DIRTY DOZEN AND THE CLEAN FIFTEEN

A nonprofit environmental watchdog organization called Environmental Working Group (EWG) looks at data supplied by the US Department of Agriculture (USDA) and the Food and Drug Administration (FDA) about pesticide residues. Each year it compiles a list of the best and worst pesticide loads found in commercial crops. You can use these lists to decide which fruits and vegetables to buy organic to minimize your exposure to pesticides and which produce is considered safe enough to buy conventionally. This does not mean they are pesticide-free, though, so wash these fruits and vegetables thoroughly.

These lists change every year, so make sure you look up the most recent one before you fill your shopping cart. You'll find the most recent lists, as well as a guide to pesticides in produce, at EWG.org/FoodNews.

Dirty Dozen

Apples
Celery
Cherries
Cherry tomatoes
Cucumbers
Grapes
Nectarines
Peaches
Spinach
Strawberries
Sweet bell peppers
Tomatoes

In addition to the Dirty Dozen, the EWG added two types of produce contaminated with highly toxic organophosphate insecticides:

Kale/Collard greens
Hot peppers

Clean Fifteen

Asparagus
Avocados
Cabbage
Cantaloupe
Cauliflower
Eggplant
Grapefruit
Honeydew Melon
Kiwis
Mangos
Onions
Papayas
Pineapples
Sweet corn
Sweet peas (frozen)

REFERENCES

American College of Cardiology/American Heart Association Task Force on Practice Guidelines. Accessed September 1, 2016. http://circ.ahajournals.org/content/early/2013/11/11/01.cir.0000437740.48606.d1

American Diabetes Association. "Age, Race, Gender, & Family History." Accessed September 10, 2016. www.diabetes.org/are-you-at-risk/lower-your-risk/nonmodifiables.html

American Dietetic Association. "Pocket Resource for Nutrition Assessment." Accessed October 1, 2016. dpg-storage.s3.amazonaws.com/dhcc/resources/PocketResources/PRNA%202009.pdf

American Kidney Fund. "Kidney Disease Statistics." Accessed October 10, 2016. www.kidneyfund.org/about-us/assets/pdfs/akf-kidneydiseasestatistics-2012.pdf

American Kidney Fund. "Kidney-Friendly Diet for CKD." Accessed November 8, 2016. www.kidneyfund.org/kidney-disease/chronic-kidney-disese-ckd/kidney-friendly-diet-for-ckd.html

American Kidney Fund. "High Potassium Hyperkalemia." Accessed November 8, 2016. www.kidneyfund.org/kidney-disease/chronic-kidney-disease-dkd/complications/high-potassium-hyperkalemia.html

Centers for Disease Control and Prevention. "National Chronic Kidney Disease Fact Sheet." Accessed October 5, 2016. www.cdc.gov/diabetes/pubs/pdf/kidney_factsheet.pdf

Clinical Journal of the American Society of Nephrology. "Prevalence of Chronic Kidney Disease in US Adults with Undiagnosed Diabetes or Prediabetes." Accessed September 30, 2016. cjasn.asnjournals.org/content/5/4/673

DaVita, Inc. "Phosphorus and Chronic Kidney Disease." Accessed October 1, 2016. www.davita.com/kidney-disease/diet-and-nutrition/diet-basics/phosphorus-and-chronic-kidney-disease/e/5306

DaVita, Inc. "Potassium and Chronic Kidney Disease." Accessed October18, 2016. www.davita.com/kidney-disease/diet-and-nutrition/diet%20basics/potassium-and-chronic-kidney-disease/e/5308

Kidney Urology Foundation of America. "High Blood Pressure and Kidney Disease." Accessed September 30, 2016. www.kidneyurology.org/Library/Kidney_Health/High_Blood_Pressure_and_Kidney_Disease.php

Krishnamurthy, V., G. Wei, B. Baird, M. Murtaugh, M. Chonchol, K. Raphael, T. Greene, and S. Beddhu. "High Dietary Fiber Intake Is Associated with Decreased Inflammation and All-Cause Mortality in Patients with Chronic Kidney Disease." *Kidney International*, 2012.

National Institute of Diabetes and Digestive and Kidney Diseases. "Eating Right for Kidney Health. Tips for People with Chronic Kidney Disease (CKD)." Accessed November 8, 2016. www.niddk.nih.gov/health-information/health-communication-programs/nkdep/a-z/eating-right/Documents/eating-right-508.pdf

National Institutes of Health. "Kidney Disease: Early Detection and Treatment." Accessed October 2, 2016. www.nlm.nih.gov/medlineplus/magazine/issues/winter08/articles/winter08pg9-10.html

The National Kidney Foundation. "Cholesterol and Chronic Kidney Disease." Accessed October 1, 2016. www.kidney.org/atoz/content/cholesterol

The National Kidney Foundation. "How Your Kidneys Work." Accessed October 1, 2016. www.kidney.org/kidneydisease/howkidneyswrk

The National Kidney Foundation. "Phosphorus and Your CKD Diet." Accessed October 1, 2016. www.kidney.org/atoz/content/phosphorus

The National Kidney Foundation. "Vitamins and Minerals in Kidney Disease." Accessed October 1, 2016. www.kidney.org/atoz/content/vitamineral

The National Kidney Foundation. "KDOQI Clinical Practice Guidelines and Clinical Practice Recommendations for Diabetes and Chronic Kidney Disease." Accessed November 1, 2016. www.kidney.org/sites/default/files/docs/diabetes-ckd-update-2012.pdf

The National Kidney Foundation. "10 Signs You Have Kidney Disease." Accessed October 1, 2016. www.kidney.org/news/ekidney/august14/10_Signs_You_May_Have_Kidney_Disease

The Renal Association. "Chronic Kidney Disease Stages." Accessed October 15, 2016. www.renal.org/information-resources/the-uk-eckd-guide/ckd-stages#sthash.jWT6jJfH.dpbs

The Renal Association. "Nutrition in CKD". Accessed November 1, 2016. www.renal.org/guidelines/modules/nutrition-in-ckd

US National Library of Medicine. "Chronic Kidney Disease." Accessed November 1, 2016. www.nlm.nih.gov/medlineplus/ency/article/000471.htm

RECIPE INDEX

INDEX

ACKNOWLEDGMENTS

First and foremost I would like to thank God. You have given me the power and strength to believe in my passion and pursue my dreams. I could never have done this without the faith I have in you.

This book would also not be possible without the many patients I've had the pleasure of working with over the many years. My passion for working in the renal community is because of you.

I would like to thank my family, especially my siblings, Marie, David, Abdo, and Tony, who always support me no matter how crazy my ideas seem to be. My sisters-in-law, Gina and Deena, I am constantly in awe of your support. My brother-in-law, Gordon, who's always rooting for me. Thank you all from the bottom of my heart.

I would like to thank Michelle Anderson, Patty Consolazio, and Therezia Alchoufete for helping me in what seems the endless process of selecting and editing.

Meg Ilasco—third time's a charm. What a pleasure it's been working with you. Thank you for believing in me.

ABOUT THE AUTHOR

Susan Zogheib was born in Beirut, Lebanon, and moved to the United States with her family in the late 1980s. She is a registered dietitian and holds a master's degree from Ryerson University in Toronto, Ontario, Canada, in nutrition communication. Susan is a food and nutrition expert and media consultant with more than ten years of experience working as a clinical and renal dietitian. She believes in keeping cooking simple, fun, and healthy. Susan is the author of *Renal Diet Cookbook* and *The Mediterranean Diet Plan*.

CPSIA information can be obtained
at www.ICGtesting.com
Printed in the USA
BVHW02s0259250818
525438BV00003B/5/P